HANDBOOK OF DIAGNOSIS AND TREATMENT OF THE DSM-IV PERSONALITY DISORDERS

HANDBOOK OF DIAGNOSIS AND TREATMENT OF THE DSM-IV PERSONALITY DISORDERS

Len Sperry, M.D., Ph.D.

BRUNNER/MAZEL *Publishers* • New York

Library of Congress Cataloging-in-Publication Data

Sperry, Len.
 Handbook of diagnosis and treatment of the DSM-IV personality disorders /
by Len Sperry
     p. cm.
 Includes bibliographical references and index.
 ISBN 0-87630-780-2
 1. Personality Disorders.   I. Title.
 [DNLM: 1. Personality Disorders—diagnosis—handbooks.
2. Personality Disorders—therapy—handbooks. 3. Personality Disorders—classification—handbooks.   WM 39 S751h 1995]
 RC554.S73   1995
 616.89—dc20
 DNLM/DLC
 for Library of Congress   94-44790
                                                                 CIP

Published by
BRUNNER/MAZEL, INC.
19 Union Square West
New York, New York 10003
Manufactured in the United States of America

10 9 8 7 6 5 4 3 2

Acknowledgments

I wish to express my appreciation to a number of people who helped make this book a reality. Various early drafts of these chapters were read by and discussed with psychiatry residents in seminars and supervision with me at the Medical College of Wisconsin. At Brunner/Mazel, Mark Tracten, Richard Sauber, Bernie Mazel, and particularly Natalie Gilman have been incredibly supportive of the idea for this book. Patricia Wolf's editorial assistance was invaluable. Finally, Dawn Stalbaum has invested much time and effort in transforming my barely legible handwriting into typewritten form. To all of these individuals go my heartfelt thanks.

This book is dedicated to Frank K. Johnson, M.D. First my residency director, and then valued colleague and friend, Frank has been a source of wise counsel and support over these past two decades.

Contents

Preface

The fact that personality disorders really exist, appear to be increasing in prevalence, and often are difficult, if not impossible, to treat has become a sobering reality for mental health professionals. Until a few years ago, clinicians were beginning to feel comfortable and competent with utilizing some of the newer, focused brief treatment methods for a variety of anxiety, depressive, and other Axis I disorders. Then along came a tidal wave of anxious and depressed individuals who were, for all practical purposes, nonresponsive to these methods—even when bolstered by medication—because of the presence of a concurrent Axis II personality disorder. Now optimism is again mounting about the treatability of personality disorders. And this optimism has inspired a search for more information on and specific skills for assessing and treating these disorders. Articles, books, and workshops on treating personality disorders are hot commodities today.

A number of professional titles on the treatment of personality disorders have been published of late. They tend to fall into one of three categories. Most of them are about specific principles and strategies for a specific personality disorder, typically borderline personality or narcissistic personality. A smaller number of books provide specific principles and strategies for all of the DSM personality disorders. Usually, they adopt a particular stance, for example: Beck, Freeman, and Associates' *Cognitive Therapy of the Personality Disorders*; Benjamin's *Interpersonal Diagnosis and Treatment of Personality Disorders*; and the section on personality disorders in Gabbard's *Psychodynamic Psychiatry in Clinical Practice*. The smallest number of titles address general principles and strategies for the various personality disorders. These tend to be edited volumes, such as that by Lion, *Personality Disorders: Diagnosis and Management*.

For the most part, these books emphasize individual psychotherapy, although research indicates that group or family therapy or a combination of formats and approaches is the treatment of choice for most individuals with personality disorders. In my 20-plus years of teaching and supervising mental health professionals, I found that clinicians were looking for a comprehensive source of treatment modalities and approaches for all the personality disorders. Thus this *Handbook of Diagnosis and Treatment of the DSM-IV Personality Disorders* is a compendium of techniques that have been shown to be effective for the various personality disorders. It focuses on ways of combining and integrating treatment modalities and approaches: individual, group, marital, and family modalities, in addition to behavioral, cognitive, interpersonal, and psychodynamic approaches and the use of medication.

Practicing clinicians in psychiatry, clinical psychology, psychiatric nursing, and mental health counseling, as well as those in training, should find specific information between the covers of this book to aid them in diagnosing personality-disordered individuals, and formulating, planning, and implementing their treatment. At least, that is my hope and expectation.

HANDBOOK OF DIAGNOSIS AND TREATMENT OF THE DSM-IV PERSONALITY DISORDERS

CHAPTER 1

Paradigm Shift in the Treatment of Personality Disorders

Mention personality disorders—particularly borderline personality disorder or antisocial personality disorder—to a colleague and you might elicit such comments as: "Most borderlines are treatment refractory," "Personality disorders have guarded prognoses at best," or "Antisocials are psychopaths and should be in prison, not psychotherapy." And what about your own reactions when a colleague wants to refer a personality-disordered individual to you? Do you feel stuck, apprehensive, or angry? Do you think about your personal safety, after-hours emergencies or telephone calls, and whether your bill will be paid?

That was how many clinicians felt about the treatment of depression as recently as 20 years ago. The therapeutic treatment of major and "minor" depression with traditional approaches did have a guarded prognosis. But today, major depression and dysthymia are highly responsive to treatment interventions and the prognoses are good to excellent. How did this happen? Essentially, a "paradigm shift" occurred in the way depression was conceptualized, assessed, and treated. A similar paradigm shift is now tak-

1

ing place in the conceptualization and assessment of the personality disorders and the relevant treatment strategies and interventions.

To understand why and how this paradigm shift is occurring with the personality disorders, it will be instructive to describe briefly the shift that took place—and is still going on—with the depressive disorders.

PARADIGM SHIFT

In the past, depression typically was conceptualized by the time-honored psychodynamic notion of anger turned inward. The first and second editions of the *Diagnostic and Statistical Manual of Mental Disorders* (DSM-I and DSM-II) described depression as a depressive reaction or neurosis attributable to an internal conflict or loss; or a psychotic depressive reaction; or manic-depressive illness, depressed type.

Today, depression is conceptualized and formulated in a number of ways. From a cognitive therapy perspective, depression results from distorted thinking, particularly negative ideas about self, the world, and the future (Beck, Rush, Shaw, & Emery, 1979). Beck called this constellation of beliefs the "cognitive triad" of depression. Behaviorists conceptualize depression as resulting from decreased experiences of pleasure (Lewinsohn, 1975). The interpersonal view is that depression is caused by interpersonal loss and conflict (Klerman & Weissman, 1984). There are a variety of contemporary psychodynamic views of depression (Arieti & Bomperad, 1978; Bellak & Siegel, 1983). For instance, Bellak and Siegel describe 10 different psychodynamic formulations. Wetzel (1984) reviews and criticizes several dynamic, cognitive, behavioral, and cultural formulations of depression from a feminist perspective. What is particularly noteworthy is that most contemporary formulations of depression—that is, psychodynamic, biological, cognitive, interpersonal—are becoming more biopsychosocially based (Sperry, Gudeman, Blackwell, & Faulkner, 1992).

In the past, DSM-I and DSM-II provided short descriptions of depressive neurosis, but offered no criteria. Assessment methods included clinical interviews, data from tests such as MMPI and their so-called "depression" scales, and the Zung Depression Inventory (Zung, 1965). Zung's instrument focused on symptoms and theoreticals. Depression might not have even been specified as a diagnosis, and clinicians, sensitive to the stigma of mental illness, often used "adjustment reaction of adulthood" instead. Because there were no agreed-upon diagnostic criteria, this practice of diagnostic minimization was common.

Today, very specific criteria and more sensitive theory-derived measures are available. DSM-III and DSM-III-R offered specific diagnostic criteria, which DSM-IV has further refined. These criteria have greatly delineated subtypes of depression, including major depressive disorder, dysthmic disorder, minor depressive disorder, and depressive personality disorder. Theoretically based self-rating instruments like the Beck Depression Inventory and clinician-rated inventories such as the Hamilton Depression Inventory are commonly used not only in research studies, but also in clinical practice. Structured interview formats have also been developed, the Schedules of Affective Disorders and Schizophrenia (SADS) being among the most common.

Treatment of depression in the past was largely expressive or supportive psychotherapy. After the release of imipramine in 1958, medication specifically targeted at depression was available, but usually was not combined with psychotherapy.

A variety of highly effective treatment interventions for the various subtypes of depression are now at hand. Many of these treatment approaches not only are theoretically based, but also are manualized, lending themselves to controlled research trials. These include cognitive therapy (Beck, 1967; Beck et al., 1979), behavior therapy (Lewinsohn et al., 1975, 1984), and interpersonal therapy of depression (Klerman & Weissman, 1984, 1993). Efforts to combine medication with various focused psychotherapies for depression have resulted in the establishment of specific treatment guidelines (Rush & Hollon, 1991). What is noticeably different about these treatment approaches is that they are highly focused and structured, and require the clinician to be rather active as compared with the traditional expressive-supportive psychotherapy of the past.

The effectiveness of some of these treatment approaches has been carefully studied. For example, outcome research, including controlled clinical trials of cognitive therapy, has demonstrated its clear efficacy against waiting list controls, as well as other focused treatments. Over 100 studies have been reported on the effectiveness of cognitive therapy.

Efforts to combine various other treatment modalities, such as medication and group therapy, individual and group therapy, and family therapy and medication, have also been described (Beitman, 1993). In addition, efforts to further increase treatment efficacy have prompted others to integrate and tailor various treatment approaches for depression, including Karasu's (1990) description of the integration of dynamic, cognitive, and interpersonal psychotherapy.

In the past, there were few preventive efforts regarding depression. Today, the highly publicized DART (Depression Awareness, Recognition, and Treatment) program appears to have effected major changes in treatment. The results of a prospective study, the San Francisco Depression Prevention Program, was recently published (Munoz & Ying, 1993). This study demonstrates that primary and secondary prevention efforts can stem the incidence of various subtypes of depression.

Why did this paradigm shift regarding the treatment of depression take place? It was largely the result of a concerted effort of clinicians, researchers, and theorists to understand its etiology and to experiment with various approaches and modalities of treatment. Now clinicians not only are quite confident that depression is treatable, but they also have been successful in their efforts to effect symptom remission and other changes with these patients.

A similar paradigm shift is occurring with regard to the conceptualization, assessment, and treatment of the personality disorders. Before 1980, personality disorders were mostly conceptualized in terms of "character language," such as anal character or obsessive character. Even though there was a biological tradition in the study of personality that emphasized temperament, the psychological tradition that emphasized character was clearly in vogue for most of the twentieth century (Stone, 1993). Descriptions of personality disorders in DSM-I and DSM-II reflected this emphasis on character and psychodynamics. Within the psychoanalytic community, character reflected specific defense mechanisms. For example, the defenses of isolation of affect, intellectualization, and rationalization were common in the obsessive-compulsive character.

Today, personality disorders are being conceptualized in a much broader fashion, which includes both character and temperament. Neurobiological and biosocial formulations of personality disorder have attracted considerable attention and have generated a considerable amount of research. Millon (1981) and Cloninger and colleagues (Cloninger, 1987; Cloninger, Svrakic, & Przybeck, 1993) hypothesize that temperament and neurotransmitters greatly influence personality development and functioning. Cloninger (Cloninger et al., 1993) describes personality as the influence of character and temperament, where temperament refers to the innate, genetic, and constitutional influences on personality, and character refers to the learned psychosocial influences. Cloninger hypothesizes that temperament has formed measurable biological subtracts—novelty seeking, harm avoidance, reward dependence, and persistence—whereas character has three quantifiable factors: self-directedness, cooperativeness, and self-transcendence. He believes that personality style reflects the individual's temperament factors plus positive or high scores on the three character factors. Conversely, personality disorders reflect negative or low scores on the three character factors.

The Five Factor Model (FFM) has become the most prominent of the contemporary psychological models of personality. Described by several authors, FFM describes personality dimensionally in terms of the factors of agreeableness, conscientiousness, neuroticism, extraversion, and openness (Costa & McCrae, 1990, 1992).

Stone (1993) discusses a "grand unified theory" of personality disorders, which basically interdigitates the FFM (a psychological model) and Cloninger's Seven Factor Model (a biosocial model). This unified theory is, essentially, a biopsychosocial theory of personality disorders. In addition to these research-based theories and models, there are a number of different clinical formulations of the personality disorders (Beck, Freeman, and Associates, 1990; Benjamin, 1993; Gabbard, 1990).

In the past, criteria for the assessment of the personality disorders were somewhat primitive. DSM-I subdivided the personality disorder into five headings: personality pattern disturbance, personality trait disturbance, sociopathic personality disturbance, special symptom reactions, and transient situational personality disorders. DSM-II, which appeared in 1968, eliminated the subheadings and streamlined the number of personality disorders. Although brief descriptions of each disorder were given, they were not based on clinical trials, and diagnostic criteria were not provided. Furthermore, no clear distinction was made between symptom disorders (Axis I) and personality disorders (Axis II).

This lack of specificity further reinforced some mistaken convictions about personality disorders. A striking example is obsessive-compulsive disorder and obsessive-compulsive personality disorder. Before DSM-III, little or no distinction was made between these disorders. Now there is consensus that the disorders have relatively little overlap (Jenike, 1991), and yet some clinicians still fail or hesitate to make this distinction, referring to both as aspects of the "obsessive personality" (Salzman, 1980). Perhaps this harkens back to Freud's case description of the Rat Man, in whom both obsessive-compulsive disorder and obsessive-compulsive personality disorder were present (Perry, Frances, & Clarkin, 1990). The implication was that both disorders are essentially the same, and so their treatment should be the same. Jenike (1991) notes that the concurrence of obsessive-compulsive personality disorder in patients with obsessive-compulsive disorder is small, probably less than 15 to 18 percent.

Previously, personality disorder was assessed by clinical interview and inferred from standardized personality inventories such as the MMPI. Today, there are a number of formal measures of the personality disorders. Some are theory and research based, such as Millon's MCMI-II (Millon, 1985) and Cloninger's Temperament Character Inventory (TCI) (Cloninger et al., 1993). Others are research-based self-report instruments, like the Personality Disorder Inventory (PDI) and the Personality Disorders Questionnaire—Revised (PDQ-R). Various semistructured schedules also are available, including the Structured Clinical Interview for DSM-III-R Personality Disorders (SCID-II). Although methodological issues have been raised about these assessment devices, they have served both the clinician and the researcher well (Zimmerman, 1994).

In large part, these assessment measures reflect the increasingly differentiated criteria of DSM-III, DSM-III-R, and DSM-IV. DSM-III subdivided 11 personality disorders—antisocial, avoidant, borderline, compulsive, dependent, histrionic, narcissistic, paranoid, passive-aggressive, schizoid, and schizotypal—into three clusters: odd, dramatic, and anxious. DSM-III-R maintained the essential features of DSM-III, but added the sadistic and self-defeating personality disorders to the appendix. DSM-IV further differentiated criteria and dropped the self-defeating and sadistic personality disorders. It relegated passive-aggressive personality disorder to the category of personality disorder not otherwise specified (NOS), as well as depressive personality disorder, which joined passive-aggressive personality disorder in Appendix B.

Formerly, the treatment of personality disorders lay largely in the domain of psychodynamic approaches. Psychoanalysis and long-term psychoanalytically oriented psychotherapy were considered the treatments of choice (Stone, 1993). The goal of treatment was to change character structure. Unfortunately, outcomes were mixed, even among patients judged amenable to treatment. For the most part, clinicians utilized a traditional exploratory approach, adopted a neutral and passive stance, and primarily employed clarification and interpretation strategies.

Treatment methods today are considerably different in that treatment tends to be more focused and structured, with the clinician taking a more active role. Many of these treatment approaches and intervention strategies are theory based and have been researched in clinical trials in comparison with other treatment approaches or other modalities, such as medication, group therapy, and family therapy. The cognitive therapy approach, the interpersonal psychotherapy approach (Benjamin, 1993), and some psychodynamic approaches have been specifically modified for the treatment of personality-disordered individuals.

Psychopharmacological research on the treatment of selected personality disorders has grown rapidly in the past eight years. Until very recently, the consensus among clinicians was that medication did not and could not treat personality disorders per se, but could be used for concurrent Axis I conditions or to target symptoms such as insomnia. This view is rapidly changing. Based on investigations of the biological correlates of personality disorders, Siever and Davis (1991) proposed a psychobiological treatment model that has been of inestimable clinical and research value. Essentially,

Siever and Davis believe that psychopharmacological treatment can and should be directed to basic dimensions that underlie the personality. These dimensions are cognitive/perceptual organizations, especially for the schizotypal and passive disorders for which low-dose antipsychotics might be useful; impulsivity and aggression in the borderline and antisocial personalities for which serotonin blockers can be useful; affective instability in borderline and histrionic personalities for which cyclic antidepressants or serotonin blockers may be useful; and anxiety/inhibition, particularly in the avoidant personalty disorder, for which serotonin blockers and monoamine oxidase inhibitor (MAOI) agents may be useful.

Consensus is growing that the effective treatment of the personality disorders involves combining treatment modalities and integrating treatment approaches. Stone (1993) suggests combining three approaches. He notes that supportive interventions, which are particularly useful in fostering a therapeutic alliance, should be augmented by psychoanalytic interventions, which are useful in resolving negative transferences at the outset of treatment, and cognitive-behavioral interventions, which are useful in the development of new attitudes and habits. Winer and Pollock (1989) and Stone (1993) also recommend combining medication with individual and group modalities for personality-disordered individuals. This prescription to integrate various approaches, as well as to combine treatment modalities, would have been considered heretical as recently as five years ago. Now the interest in integrating and combining treatments reflects an emerging consensus of opinion that underscores the immensity of the paradigm shift that is taking place.

In the past, few formal efforts were made to prevent personality disorders. This situation has not changed. However, given the efficacy of developing tertiary preventive interventions, it is conceivable that primary and secondary preventive efforts will be forthcoming.

BASIC PREMISES ABOUT THE CONTEMPORARY TREATMENT OF PERSONALITY DISORDERS

The paradigm shift in clinicians' attitudes and practice styles regarding depressive disorders and personality disorders was discussed in terms of breakthroughs, conceptualizations, assessment, and treatment. The basic premises of this book are based on these same four dimensions.

Premise 1: Personality disorders are best conceptualized in integrative and biopsychosocial terms, and the more effective treatment will reflect this biopsychosocial perspective.

Viewing personality disorders simply from a psychosocial or characterological perspective has serious limitations (Stone, 1993). Similarly, viewing personality disorders as basically biological or temperamental is also limiting. Conversely, there is considerable research and clinical support for looking at personality disorders from the perspective of character and temperament. Such a biopsychosocial or integrative clinical formulation should be reflected in a treatment plan that is biopsychosocially focused.

Premise 2: Assessing treatability or amenability to treatment is critical to maximizing treatment planning and outcomes.

Treatability is a function of a patient's readiness and level of functioning. Patient readiness refers to the individual patient's motivation for treatment and expectations for treatment outcomes, as well as past history of treatment compliance, and success, with efforts to change habits and behavior patterns. Level of functioning can be operationalized in terms of the Global Assessment of Functioning Scale (GAF) of Axis IV. High functioning refers to a score of about 65. Moderate functioning refers to scores of 45 to 65. Low functioning refers to scores below 45.

Stone (1993) suggests that personality disorders lend themselves to a three-category classification with regard to treatability: (1) high amenability, which includes the dependent, histrionic, obsessive-compulsive, avoidant, and depressive personality disorders; (2) intermediate amenability, which includes narcissistic, borderline, and schizotypal personality disorders; and (3) low amenability, which includes paranoid, passive-aggressive, schizoid, and antisocial personality disorders. Stone adds that since patients show mixtures of various personality traits, prognosis largely depends on the degree to which traits of the disorders in the third category are present. It will also depend in part on the prominence of the psychobiological dimensions described by Siever and Davis (1991): cognitive/perceptual disorganization, impulsivity/aggression, and affective inability or anxiety/inhibition. To the extent that such dimensions as impulsivity or anxiety respond to medication, concurrent psychosocial intervention efforts should be facilitated.

Premise 3: The lower the level of treatability, the more the combining and integrating of treatment modalities and approaches is needed.

Interest in combined therapies and integrative treatment has been increasing. This follows a long period in which clinicians were skeptical about, or even hostile to, combining two modalities such as individual psychotherapy and group therapy or medication and psychoanalytic psychotherapy. However, research and clinical practice reveal several advantages for combined therapeutic modalities. These include additive and even synergistic treatment effects, the dilution of unworkably intense transference relationships, and rapid symptom relief (Frances, Clarkin, & Perry 1984). Tailoring refers to modifying or adapting a particular modality or therapeutic approach to the patient's needs, style, and expectations.

A sartorial analogy might help distinguish combining, integrating, and tailoring. A man might go into a clothing store to purchase a gray business suit. He could choose a suit from the rack randomly, and there would be a small chance that it would fit perfectly, but it is more likely that it would be a poor fit. The man, whose size is usually 38 short, could look through the racks and try on a 38 short, which might fit quite well, but need some minor alterations by a tailor (partial tailoring). Of course, the person could also go to a store for a fitting and have a suit custom-made (total tailoring). Now the suit could be pure wool or pure silk, or it could be a blend of wool and silk. This blending of fabrics would be analogous to integrating treatment. Analogous to combining treatment would be purchasing a blue sports jacket that might be worn with the pants of the gray suit for a more casual look.

In short, combined treatment refers to adding modalities, such as individual, group, couple, or family, either concurrently or sequentially, while integrative treatment refers to the blending of different treatment approaches or orientations, such as psychodynamic, cognitive, behavioral, or interpersonal. Combining treatment modalities is also referred to as multimodal treatment. Finally, tailored treatment refers to specific ways of customizing treatment modalities or therapeutic approaches to "fit" the unique needs, cognitive and emotional styles, and treatment expectations of the patient.

Once considered controversial, psychoanalytically oriented therapy combined with other modalities is now being advocated by dynamically oriented clinicians. Winer and Pollack (1989) indicate that combined treatment (insight-oriented individual sessions with medication, group, or family therapy) is particularly valuable in cases of personality disorder.

Treatment delivered in combination can have an additive, and sometimes synergistic, effect. It is becoming more evident that different treatment approaches are differentially effective in resolving different types of symptom clusters. For example, in major depression, medication is more effective in remitting vegetative symptoms, whereas psychotherapy is better at improving interpersonal relationships and cognitive symptoms (Frances et al., 1984). Furthermore, the additive effect of medication and psychotherapy has been established for both major depression (Rush & Hollon, 1991) and agoraphobia (Greist & Jefferson, 1992).

What are the indications and contraindications for these various modalities? A working knowledge of these is probably more necessary for the treatment of personality disorders than with Axis I disorders. Frances, Clarkin and Perry (1984) detail the relative indications, relative contraindications, and enabling factors for three treatment modalities— individual, group, and family/marital. The reader is referred to their excellent discussion and summary table.

These authors also discuss a very basic question that needs to be asked every time a clinician considers offering treatment to a personality-disordered individual: Is treatment advisable, or would no treatment be the preferred recommendation? The "no treatment option" may be the choice for individuals who have had negative therapeutic reactions or have made little or no progress in the course of interminable therapy.

Frances et al. (1984) offer specific criteria for recommending treatment or no treatment. They also note that their research shows that patients are 10 times more likely to initiate "no treatment" decisions than are clinicians to offer it.

Whereas combined treatment refers to combining different modalities of treatment (i.e., individual and group, marital and family therapy, day treatment and inpatient treatment) either concurrently or sequentially, integrating or tailoring treatment is different. Integrative treatment refers to blending various treatment approaches (i.e., psychodynamic, cognitive, behavioral, interpersonal, and medication). Several recent publications have advocated integrative treatment for the borderline personality disorder (Stone, 1992; Linehan, 1993). Cognitive-behavioral therapy represents the integration of two therapeutic approaches: cognitive therapy and behavior therapy. The specific type of cognitive-behavioral therapy developed by Linehan, dialectical behavior therapy, is an integration of various cognitive-behavioral intervention strategies and Zen practice (Heard & Linehan, 1994). Stone (1992) prescribes blending psychoanalytic, behavioral, cognitive, and medication interventions or approaches.

If the patient's treatability is high (i.e., level of functioning and treatment readiness), the less immediate will be the need to combine and blend most of the modalities and approaches. The lower the functioning, the more modalities and approaches will need to be combined and blended.

This premise may seem quite demanding of the clinician's professional resources. And it is. Not every clinician is suited for working with all personality-disordered individuals, particularly those with low amenability to treatment. Specialized training and supervision in the utilization of various approaches are needed in the treatment of the personality disorders. It is not suggested that clinicians should or must also be trained in the various treatment modalities. Obviously, referral to group or family therapy or other treatment modalities beyond the clinician's competence is a reasonable option.

Premise 4: The basic goal of treatment is to facilitate movement from personality-disordered functioning to personality-style functioning.

Treatment goals can be thought of in terms of levels. The first level involves symptoms. The second level involves personality features that are related to environment and are modifiable. The third level involves personality features that are related to character. The fourth level involves personality functions related to temperament. Treatment of levels 1 and 2 is relatively straightforward. Medication or behavioral treatments such as exposure may quickly remit symptoms of personality. Psychotherapeutic interventions of various approaches and modalities can often be useful at level 3, but also may not be, as in the case of rule-breaking behavior of the antisocial individual. Level 4 is temperament, and human nature is not easily changed.

Stone (1993) uses the analogy of the cabinet maker and carpenter to describe this last level of treatment. The clinician working with personality-disordered individuals is not a carpenter who rebuilds a structure, but is rather like the cabinet maker who sands it down and takes the rough edges off. The temperament remains, but with treatment, the individual becomes a person with whom it is somewhat easier to work or live. Essentially then, personality style will be used in the subsequent chapters to refer to highly adaptive functioning behavior for a particular personality type, whereas personality disorder refers to functioning that is characterized by specific DSM-IV diagnostic criteria.

CHAPTER OUTLINE

Chapters 2 through 12 follow the same general format or chapter outline as noted in Table 1.1.

Each chapter is divided into five major sections: overview, description, clinical formulations, assessment, and treatment. The overview section provides a brief historical sketch of the disorder, including its evolution in DSM. It also reports incidence/prevalence data on the disorder.

The section on description provides an extensive discussion of the particular personality disorder in biopsychosocial terms. Emphasized are such aspects of temperament as cognitive style, emotional style, behavioral style, and interpersonal style. To assist the clinician in establishing whether the presentation is one of disorder or style and in deciding what the profile of

Table 1.1
Chapter Format

I.   Overview and Background
II. Characteristic Features
     1. Description
         a. Behavioral
         b. Cognitive
         c. Emotional
         d. Interpersonal
     2. Style Versus Disorder
     3. DSM-IV Criteria
III. Formulations
     1. Psychodynamic
     2. Biosocial
     3. Cognitive-Behavioral
     4. Interpersonal
     5. Integrative
IV. Assessment
     1. Interview Behavior and Rapport
     2. Psychological Testing Data
         a. MMPI-2
         b. MCMI-II
         c. TAT/Rorschach
V.   Treatment Approaches and Interventions
     1. Individual Psychotherapy
         a. Psychodynamic: Long Term and Short Term
         b. Cognitive-Behavioral
         c. Interpersonal
     2. Group Therapy
     3. Marital/Family Therapy
     4. Medication
     5. Combined/Integrative Approaches and Interventions

successful treatment of the disorder would look like, criteria and case examples of both the personality style and disorder are provided. Finally, the DSM-IV description and criteria are listed. Psychiatric formulation can be thought of in terms of descriptive, explanatory, and treatment formulations (Sperry, Gudeman, Blackwell, & Faulkner, 1992). This section represents a descriptive formulation of the disorder.

The next section contains five different explanatory conceptualizations of the disorder. The four dominant contemporary formulations are psychodynamic: the biosocial, represented largely by Millon (1981, 1990); the cognitive, represented largely by Beck et al. (1990); the behavioral, represented by Turkat (1990); and the interpersonal, described by Benjamin (1993). The fifth category is the integrative or biopsychosocial, developed by Sperry (1990) and Sperry and Mosak (1993) based on Alfred Adler's view of neurosis (Adler, 1964).

The section on assessment describes typical interview behavior exhibited by the personality-disordered patient and the ease or difficulty of establishing rapport. It also describes characteristic response patterns common for this personality disorder on such psychological tests as the MMPI-I; the MCMI-II, which is based on Millon's (1981, 1990) biosocial formulation and research data; and two common projective tests, the Rorschach and the Therapeutic Apperception Test (TAT). Since psychological testing can be particularly useful in clarifying a dimensional characterization of the patient's personality (i.e., where more than one personality disorder or cluster of traits is present), this section may be clinically relevant to psychologists and others who utilize psychological assessment.

The last section contains a number of treatment formulations, and perhaps is the most clinically useful. Beginning with a list of typical Axis I and Axis II disorders in the differential diagnosis, other treatment considerations, such as general treatment goals and strategies, are highlighted.

The three general approaches most commonly utilized in the individual treatment of the disorder are detailed: the psychodynamic, the cognitive-behavioral, and the interpersonal. The psychodynamic approaches usually include a description of the ways in which the traditional analytic method has been modified for this disorder in expressive-supportive terms. Beck et al. (1990) cognitive therapy of personality disorder approach is highlighted, and complemented with the research-based behavioral approach of Turkat (1990). Benjamin's (1993) protocol for interpersonal treatment also is presented.

Other modalities of treatment relevant to the disorder are explored, along with the related research on theory indications and efficacy. A unique feature of this book is the discussion of group, marital and family, and psychopharmacology modalities for each disorder. The group treatment modality can be either homogeneous or heterogeneous, and structured and time limited or less structured and ongoing. Heterogeneous refers to the composition of the group as diverse in terms of functioning. Homogeneous refers to the group members as being similar in terms of personality types and level of functioning (Frances et al., 1984). Homogeneous groups lend themselves to being structured and time limited. Finally, specific suggestions for combining modalities and integrating or blending treatment approaches round out this section and the book. Because the borderline and narcissistic personality disorders have been the most widely discussed and studied, those two chapters are the most extensive in terms of treatment protocols.

CONCLUDING NOTE

A paradigm shift is occurring in the treatment of the personality disorders, which will require a major change in the way clinicians conceptualize, assess, and treat these disorders. This change in attitude and practice patterns will be resisted by those who find the prospect of combining and blending modalities and approaches, or of taking a more structured and active role in the treatment process, either heretical or threatening, or both. For most others, the challenge and prospects of the future make the change a necessity. It has even been suggested that although personality-disordered patients may not respond as easily and as quickly as depressed patients, they "may become our most welcome clients in the new century, clients who are deeply troubled, but whom we can help with confidence" (*Clinical Psychiatry News*, 1991).

CHAPTER 2

Antisocial Personality Disorder

In the past, those with antisocial personality disorders were called psychopaths, sociopaths, or dyssocial personalities. Descriptions of antisocial personality can be traced to early Greek literature. It was the prototypical personality disorder, in that the term "psychopath" originally referred to
personality disorders in general. The psychopathic personality as described
by Cleckley (1941) included superficial charm, unreliability, poor judgment,
and a lack of social responsibility, guilt, anxiety, and remorse. This term
was replaced by "sociopath" to reflect the social rather than purely psychological origins of the disorder. In DSM-II, antisocial personality became
the preferred designation. DSM-III added detailed diagnostic criteria for
this diagnosis, which largely emphasized criminal activity and behavior.
Dynamically oriented clinicians criticized the criteria for disregarding
psychodynamic qualities, such as incapacity for love, failure to learn from
experience, and lack of shame or remorse. DSM-III-R responded to such
criticism by adding the criterion "lacks remorse." Changes in DSM-IV criteria are notable for their emphasis on psychopathic traits and deemphasis
on criminal behaviors (Widiger & Corbitt, 1993; Gabbard, 1994).

15

Overall prevalence of this disorder is about 3 percent for men and 1 percent for women. In clinical settings, prevalence estimates vary from 3 to 30 percent, with higher rates associated with prisons, forensic settings, and substance abuse treatment programs.

This chapter describes the characteristic features of the antisocial personality disorder and its related personality style. Five clinical formulations of the disorder and psychological assessment indicators are highlighted. A variety of treatment approaches, modalities, and intervention strategies are also described.

CHARACTERISTICS OF THE ANTISOCIAL PERSONALITY STYLE AND DISORDER

Antisocial personalities can be thought of as spanning a continuum from healthy to pathological, wherein the antisocial personality style is at the healthy end and the antisocial personality disorder is at the pathological end. Table 2.1 compares and contrasts the antisocial personality style and disorder.

The antisocial personality disorder can be recognized by the following behavior and interpersonal, cognitive, and emotional styles.

The behavioral style of antisocial personalities is characterized by impulsivity, irritability, and aggressiveness. They are likely to be irresponsible in honoring work commitments and financial obligations. Rule breaking is typical. Persons with antisocial personality disorders are also noted for their impulsive anger, deceitfulness, and cunning. They tend to be forceful individuals who regularly engage in risk- and thrill-seeking behavior.

Their interpersonal style is characterized by antagonism and a reckless disregard of others' needs and safety. They tend to be highly competitive and distrustful of others, and are often poor losers. In their relationships, they may appear at times to be "slick," as well as calculating. These behaviors can characterize the successful businessperson, politician, and professional, as well as the criminal. These individuals tend to develop superficial relationships that involve few, if any, lasting emotional ties or commitments. Furthermore, they tend to be callous about the pain and suffering of others.

The cognitive style of antisocial personality is described as impulsive and cognitively inflexible, as well as externally oriented. These individual tend to be keenly aware of social cues and may be quite adept at "reading" people and situations. Because they are contemptuous of authority, rules, and social norms, they easily rationalize their own behavior. Impulsivity, irritability, and aggressivity predispose them to argumentation, and even assaultive action.

Table 2.1.
A Comparison of Features of the Antisocial Personality Style and Disorder

Personality Style	Personality Disorder
• Prefer free-lancer living, and live-well behavior.	• Unable to sustain consistent work by their talents, skills, ingenuity, or wits.
• Tend to live by their own internal code of values and are not much influenced by others or society's norms.	• Fail to conform to social norms with regard to lawful behavior, performing antisocial acts that are grounds for arrest (rule breaking).
• As adolescents were usually high-spirited hell-raisers and mischief makers.	• Irritable and aggressive, as indicated by physical fights or assaults.
• Tend to be generous with money, believing that as it is spent, more will turn up somewhere and somehow.	• Repeatedly fail to honor financial obligations.
• Tend to have wanderlust, but are able to make plans and commitments, albeit for limited time spans.	• Fail to plan ahead or are impulsive, as indicated by moving about without a prearranged job or clear goals.
• Tend to be silver-tongued, gifted in the art of winning friends.	• Have no regard for the truth, as indicated by repeated lying, use of aliases, or "conning" others for personal profit or pleasure.
• Tend to be courageous, physically bold, and tough; will stand up to those who dare take to advantage of them.	• Reckless disregard of their own and others' personal safety, as indicated by driving while intoxicated or recurrent speeding.
• Tend not to worry too much about others, expecting others to be responsible for themselves.	• If parents or guardians, lack the ability to function as responsible parents.
• Have strong libidos, and while they may desire others, can remain monogamous for long periods.	• Have never sustained a totally monogamous relationship for more than one year.
• Tend to live in the present and do not feel much guilt.	• Lack remorse (feel justified in having hurt, mistreated, or stolen from others).

Their feelings or emotional style is characterized as shallow and superficial. They avoid "softer" emotions such as warmth and intimacy, because they regard these as signs of weakness. Guilt is seldom, if ever, experienced. They are unable to tolerate boredom, depression, or frustration, and so are sensation seekers. Finally, they may show little guilt, shame, or remorse for their own deviant actions.

The following two cases further illustrate the differences between the antisocial personality disorder (Juan G.) and the antisocial personality style (Gordon J.).

Case Study: Antisocial Personality Disorder

Juan G. is a 28-year-old man who presented late in the evening to the emergency room at a community hospital complaining of a headache. His description of the pain was vague and contradictory. At one point, he said the pain had been present for three days, whereas at another point, he said it was "many years." He indicated that the pain led to violent behavior, and described how, during a headache episode, he had brutally assaulted a medic while he was in the Air Force. He gave a long history of arrests for assault, burglary, and drug dealing. The results of neurological and mental status examinations were within normal limits, except for some mild agitation. He insisted that only Darvon, a narcotic, would relieve his headache pain. The patient resisted a plan for further diagnostic tests or a follow-up clinic appointment, saying that unless he was treated immediately, "something really bad could happen."

Case Study: Antisocial Personality Style

Gordon J. is the 38-year-old president of a rapidly expanding manufacturing company. After assuming management of the small business founded by his uncle following World War II, he had greatly increased production, had added new product lines, and had formed a marketing and sales group that he personally supervised in the nine years he had been running the firm. Prior to taking over the company, Gordon had worked for three years for a real estate firm, where he had become the youngest member of the million-dollar sales club. His father had died in a freak skiing accident when Gordon was 11 years old, but that did not stop Gordon from pursuing his own fascination with scuba diving and hang-glider flying. Gordon was invited to join the Young Presidents Organization (YPO) in his region soon after turning his uncle's corporation into a highly profitable enterprise. He was quite popular in the group, given his magnetic personality, visionary outlook, and captivating stories of his various exploits. He had been married for nearly five years before divorcing. Since then, he has not remarried, but has maintained ongoing relationships with two women.

DSM-IV Description and Criteria

Persons with antisocial personality disorders when in an out-of-therapy situation are likely to be impulsive, deceitful, and irresponsible, and rule benders and breakers. Table 2.2 gives the DSM-IV clinical description and criteria.

FORMULATIONS OF THE ANTISOCIAL PERSONALITY DISORDER

Psychodynamic Formulation

Psychoanalytic writers describe antisocial personality as similar to the narcissistic personality. While both form a pathological grandiose self, the an-

Table 2.2.
DSM-IV Criteria for Antisocial Personality Disorder*

301.7 Antisocial Personality Disorder

A. There is a pervasive pattern of disregard for and a violation of the rights of others occurring since age 15 years, as indicated by three (or more) of the following:

   (1) failure to conform to social norms with respect to lawful behaviors as indicated by repeatedly performing acts that are grounds for arrest

   (2) deceitfulness, as indicated by repeated lying, use of aliases, or conning others for personal profit or pleasure

   (3) impulsivity or failure to plan ahead

   (4) irritability and aggressiveness, as indicated by repeated physical fights or assaults

   (5) reckless disregard for safety of self or others

   (6) consistent irresponsibility, as indicated by repeated failure to sustain consistent work behavior or honor financial obligations

   (7) lack of remorse, as indicated by being indifferent to or rationalizing having hurt, mistreated, or stolen from another

B. The individual is at least age 18 years.

C. There is evidence of Conduct Disorder with onset before age 15 years.

D. The occurrence of antisocial behavior is not exclusively during the course of Schizophrenia or a Manic Episode.

*Reprinted with permission from the *Diagnostic and Statistical Manual of Mental Disorders, Fourth Edition.* Copyright 1994 American Psychiatric Association.

tisocial individual's self is based on an aggressive introject, called the "stranger self-object" (Meloy, 1988). This self-object reflects an experience of the parent as a stranger who could not be trusted and who harbored bad will toward the infant. Not surprisingly, this threatening internalized object derives from experiences of parental neglect or cruelty. Combined with the absence of a loving maternal object is a lack of basic trust and a fixation in the separation–individuation process so that object constancy does not occur. Since the mother is experienced as a stranger or predator, the infant's emotional attachment to her is derailed, leading to a detachment from all relationships and affective experiences, as well as sadistic attempts to bond with others through destructive and controlling behaviors.

As a result, antisocial individuals do not perceive others as separate individuals, hence cannot develop a capacity for guilt and depressive anxieties based on how their actions hurt others. A corollary is that they are incapable of true depression. Kernberg (1984) notes that these antisocial individuals are similarly stunted in superego development, except for sadistic superego precursors made manifest by cruel and sadistic behaviors. More highly functioning antisocial individuals are noted to have some development of consciousness within circumscribed areas—called superego lacunae—where their superegos do not seem to function. Furthermore, antisocial individuals show little interest in rationalizing or morally justifying their behavior or in adhering to a value system other than the exploitive, aggressive exercise of power (Kernberg, 1984; Meloy, 1988).

Biosocial Formulation

There is mounting evidence that biological factors influence the development of antisocial personality. Low levels of the neurotransmitter serotonin have been noted in individuals prone to aggressive and impulsive behavior. Meloy (1988) suggests that antisocial individuals often have histories of childhood abuse or neglect. They are likely to have had a "difficult infant" temperament (Thomas & Chess, 1977), meaning that they were difficult to soothe and comfort. This may have interfered with the normal attachment process, further increasing the probability of childhood abuse or neglect. Millon and Everly (1985) suggest that low thresholds for limbic system stimulation are likely in antisocial individuals. Meloy (1988) adds that they have been found to be autonomically hyperactive, possibly because of their inability to learn from experience, and thus entertain less anticipatory anxiety to deter them from ill-advised behavior.

Environmental factors such as parental hostility, deficient parental role modeling, and reinforcement of vindictive behavior appear to interact with these biological predisposing factors. Parental hostility may result from the child's disruptiveness, from the perception that these children are ill-tempered, or because they are used as scapegoats for the parents' or family's frustration. Deficient parental modeling results when there is little or no parental guidance or there is no authority figure in the home. Without an authority figure to model, and feeling abandoned or rejected, these children often become streetwise and hardened to the world around them. Out of these experiences, they learn that "the end justifies the means," that "it's a dog-eat-dog world," and that "you've got to be strong and crafty to survive." Not surprisingly, this defiant behavior is met with social disapproval, which further reinforces their self-reliance and hardened outlook. As a result, they learn not to trust others, and anticipating that others will try to exploit or humiliate them, they strike out with vindictive behaviors.

This personality pattern is self-perpetuated through consistent perceptual distortion, a demeaning attitude toward affection and cooperation, and antagonism and vindictive behavior that breeds antagonism in return. Further, this pattern is perpetuated by their fear of being used and forced into an inferior, dominated position (Millon & Everly, 1985).

Cognitive-Behavioral Formulations

According to Beck et al. (1990), the behavior of an individual with antisocial personality disorder is guided by a number of self-serving dysfunctional cognitions. These frequently include justification, or the belief that wanting something or wanting to avoid something justifies one's actions; thinking is believing, or the belief that one's thoughts and feelings are always accurate; personal inflexibility, or the belief that one's choices are invariably right and good; feelings make facts, or the belief that one is right because one feels right about one's actions; or the belief that others' views are irrelevant to one's decisions; and low-impact consequences, or the belief that undesirable consequences will not occur or will not matter. Underlying these dysfunctional cognitions are beliefs about the self and the world. Antisocial individuals tend to view themselves as loners, as autonomous and strong. They view life as harsh and cruel and others as either exploitative and manipulative or as weak and vulnerable. Accordingly, they believe that they must look out for themselves, and they adopt the strategy of overtly attacking others, or of "conning" them by subtly manipulating or exploiting them. Another core belief is that the antisocial individual is always right, which absolves the person from questioning his or her own actions. Similarly, because of their mistrust, antisocial individuals are unlikely to seek the advice or guidance of others regarding their past, present, or anticipated actions. Furthermore, they are likely to dismiss unsolicited counsel from others as irrelevant to their purposes. Finally, antisocial individuals are oriented only to the present, eschewing any concern for future outcomes.

Evans and Sullivan (1990) found that several thinking errors or manipulative strategies characterize antisocial individuals. These include mind reading, minimizing, excuse making, blaming, superoptimism, vagueness, making power plays, lying, intellectualizing, and excitement seeking. Turkat (1990) describes three subtypes: the clear sociopath, meaning one who clearly and obviously meets DSM-III-R criteria; the clever sociopath, who feigns psychological symptoms, usually to avoid legal responsibility for his or her actions; and the hurting sociopath, who meets the DSM criteria but is sincerely and genuinely distressed. He observes that all three types have deficits regarding the management of impulses and anger, but that only the hurting sociopath is somewhat amenable to treatment.

Interpersonal Formulation

For Benjamin (1993), persons with antisocial personality disorders typically have developmental histories of harsh, neglectful parenting. The adult consequence of this is that the antisocial individual neglects and is insensitive to the needs of others or exploits others. The unpredictable pattern of parenting tends to result in undermodulated parental control and blaming. The result is that, as adults, antisocial individuals fiercely protect their autonomy. Furthermore, this pattern of inept parental caring can be internalized by the antisocial individual and result in substance abuse, criminal behavior, or parental dereliction of duty. The antisocial-to-be is likely to "take over" parental responsibilities, since no one else did. As a consequence of this inappropriate parental role taking, the antisocial individual is likely to continue controlling others as an end in itself, without emotionally bonding with those being controlled. In short, a sustained pattern of inappropriate and unmodulated desire for control of others is prominent. There is also a strong need for independence, and to resist being controlled by others, who typically are held in contempt. Unbridled aggressivity is frequently utilized to sustain control and independence. Finally, antisocial-disordered individuals may present as friendly and sociable, albeit in a somewhat detached manner, since they have little regard for others.

Integrative Formulation

The following integrative formulation may be helpful in understanding how antisocial personality developed and is maintained. Biologically, antisocial personalities had exhibited "difficult child" temperaments (Thomas & Chess, 1977). As such, they were unpredictable, tended to withdraw from situations, were highly intense, and had a fairly low, discontented mood. This ill-tempered infantile pattern has been described by Millon (1981) as resulting, in part, from a low threshold for limbic stimulation and a decrease in the inhibitory centers of the central nervous system. Their body types tend to be endomorphic (thin and frail) or mesomorphic (athletic) (Millon, 1981).

Psychologically, their views of themselves, others, the world, and life's purpose can be articulated in terms of the following themes. They tend to view themselves with some variant of the theme: "I am cunning and entitled to get whatever I want." In other words, they see themselves as strong, competitive, energetic, and tough. Their view of life and the world is a variant of the theme: "Life is devious and hostile, and rules keep me from fulfilling my needs." Not surprisingly, their life's goal is a variant of the theme: "Therefore, I'll bend or break these rules because my needs come first, and I'll defend against efforts to be controlled or degraded by others." Acting out and rationalization are common defense mechanisms used by the antisocial personality.

Socially, predictable parenting styles and environmental factors can be noted for the antisocial personality disorder. Typically, the parenting style is characterized by hostility and deficient parental modeling. Or the parents might have provided such good modeling that the child could not or refused to live up to the high parental standards. The parental injunction is, "The end justifies the means." Thus vindictive behavior is modeled and reinforced. The family structure tends to be disorganized and disengaged. The antisocial pattern is confirmed, reinforced, and perpetuated by the following individual and systems factors: the need to be powerful and the fear of being abused and humiliated, leading to a denial of "softer" emotions plus uncooperativeness. This, along with the tendency to provoke others, leads to further reinforcement of antisocial beliefs and behaviors (Sperry & Mosak, 1993).

ASSESSMENT OF THE ANTISOCIAL PERSONALITY DISORDER

Several sources of information are useful in establishing a diagnosis and treatment plan for personality disorders. Observation, collateral information, and psychological testing are important adjuncts to the patient's self-report in the clinical interview. This section briefly describes some characteristic observations that the clinician makes and the nature of the rapport likely to develop in initial encounters with specific personality-disordered individuals. Characteristic response patterns on various objective (i.e., MMPI-2 and MCMI-II) and projective (i.e., Rorschach and TAT) tests are also described.

Table 2.3
Characteristics of Antisocial Personality Disorder

1. Behavior appearance	Impulsively angry, hostile, cunning; forceful, risk taking, thrill seeking; temper, verbally or physically abusive; avoids "softer" emotion such as warmth and intimacy, considering them weakness
2. Interpersonal behavior	Antagonistic to belligerent considering them "slick" but calculating; highly competitive and poor loser; distrustful of others
3. Cognitive style	Impulsive, inflexible, and externally oriented; hard nosed, realistic, and devious; defense is acting out
4. Feeling style	Glib, shallow, superficial
5. Parental injunction/environment	"The end justifies the means." Parental hostility—learned vindictive behavior (+) deficient authority figure; disorganized family and/or subculture system
6. Biological/temperament	Ill-tempered infantile pattern; low threshold for limbic stimulation and inefficient inhibitory centers (+); mesomorphic–endomorphic body types (subclass) adult ADD—residual
7. Self view	"I'm cunning and I'm entitled to get what I want." Views self as strong, competitive, self-reliant, energetic, and tough
8. World view	"Life is devious and hostile, and rules keep me from fulfilling my needs. Therefore, I'll bend or break them because my needs come first, and I'll defend any efforts to be controlled or degraded."
9. Self and system perpetuant	Needs to be powerful (+) fear of being abused/humiliated→ denial of tender feelings and unwillingness to cooperate (+) tendency to provoke others→ reinforcement of antisocial style

Interviewing individuals with antisocial personality disorders can be particularly challenging. Although it is easy to communicate with them as long as the clinician plays along, they become angry and critical when the clinician resists their manipulations. It is very difficult to get them to focus on their impulsivity, their irresponsibility, or the negative consequences of their actions. This lack of genuineness and sincerity limits rapport. Nevertheless, these individuals crave attention, and the clinician can stimulate discussion by encouraging them to display their accomplishments. By avoiding a judgmental or accusatory tone, the clinician may be able to encourage cooperation and help them to explore the negative consequences of their actions. When they are unwilling to cooperate or to answer questions, or they adopt complaining or hostile postures, the clinician will do well to display indifference or to initiate termination of the interview. Both of these strategies may quickly reverse their behavior. However, while they are seldom remorseful about their deceit and mistreatment of others, they can be made to realize that things are going poorly for them and that they are ruining their lives. The clinician can establish rapport and review their difficulties free of distortions and lies by showing empathy for the consequences of their behavior and failures. Only when they perceive the clinician as a nonpunitive ally who will support their constructive goals and who shows an understanding of their inability to follow social forms, can they begin to form a therapeutic alliance (Othmer & Othmer, 1989).

The Minnesota Multiphasic Personality Inventory (MMPI-2), the Millon Clinical Multiaxial Inventory (MCMI-II), the Rorschach Psychodiagnostic Test, and the Thematic Apperception Test (TAT) can be useful in diagnosing antisocial personality style or trait.

On the MMPI-2, the 4–9/9–4 (Psychopathic Deviant–Hypomania) profile is considered the classic profile of the antisocial personality disorder. Whereas the 9 represents the activator energizer of acting-out behavior, the 4 represents the cognitive component of the psychopathy. Two patterns of antisocial personality or psychopathology have been noted (Megargee & Bohn, 1979). The primary psychopath is easily provoked to violence, and thus a spike on scale 4 (Psychopathic Deviant), with elevations on 6 (Paranoid) and 8 (Schizophrenia), is likely. The 4–9/9–4 profile is more suggestive of secondary psychopathy, as is the 2–4/4–2 (Depression—Psychopathic Deviant) profile (Meyer, 1993).

On the MCMI-II, elevations on scale 5 (Narcissistic) and 6A (Antisocial) are most likely. Because alcohol and drug abuse are common in antisocial individuals, elevations in B (Alcohol Dependence) and T (Drug Dependence) are expected. Since antisocial individuals are usually not highly distressed, elevations on A (Anxiety), D (Dysthymia), and H (Somatoform) are not common.

Projective techniques can be very helpful in assessing the antisocial patient's object relations and superego development. Although patients are more likely to deceive a clinician during a clinical interview by simulating guilt or remorse, they are less likely to do so with ambiguous stimuli such as Rorschach blots where there are no "correct" answers (Gabbard, 1994).

On the Rorschach, antisocial individuals tend to produce only a low to average number of responses, and they even reject cards that they clearly could handle cognitively. There is often a delayed reaction to the color cards, but then they may respond with C (Pure Color) responses in a fairly primitive and impulsive manner. They tend to give a high number of A (Animal) and P (Popular) responses, and a low number of M (Human Movement) and W (Whole) responses. An absence of shading (Y, YF, and FY) and a low number of Form-plus (F+%) responses is noted (Wagner & Wagner, 1981).

On the TAT, their stories tend to be juvenile and sophomoric. And although the protagonist may be caught in a negative act, there is usually no mention of the consequences of that act (Bellak, 1993).

TREATMENT APPROACHES AND INTERVENTIONS

Treatment Considerations

This diagnosis is reserved for individuals over the age of 18 who have a history of symptoms of conduct disorder before the age of 15. The designation of adult antisocial behavior is used to describe criminal, aggressive, or other antisocial behavior that does not fully meet the criteria for antisocial personality disorder.

The differential diagnosis of antisocial personality disorder includes other Axis II personality disorders, such as the narcissistic personality disorder and the paranoid personality disorder. The most common Axis I syndromes associated with antisocial personality disorder are substance abuse and dependence, acute anxiety states, delusional disorders, and factitious disorders.

In terms of treatment goals, there is a consensus that the prognosis is guarded with most treatment modalities, unless the specific patient attributes are present (i.e., core depressive features). Typically, these individuals are not interested in treatment or are refractory to treatment if it is made compulsory by employees, family members, or the courts (Reid, 1989).

INDIVIDUAL PSYCHOTHERAPIES

This section reviews the psychodynamic, cognitive-behavioral, and interpersonal approaches of individual psychotherapy with individuals with antisocial personality disorders.

Psychodynamic Psychotherapy Approach

There is relatively little literature on successful treatment outcomes of individual dynamic psychotherapy with persons with antisocial personality disorders. In fact, there is widespread pessimism as to whether dynamic psychotherapy can change the antisocial pattern (Vaillant & Perry, 1985). A number of explanations have been offered for this seeming failure. They involve both patient selection and therapeutic stance and interventions.

Gabbard (1990) indicates that the clinician's task at the outset of treatment is to determine which patients are "worth" the time, energy, and money required by a long-term therapy process with an uncertain outcome. Meloy (1988) has identified the five following contraindications to psychotherapy with antisocial patients: a history of sadistic, violent behavior toward others; total absence of remorse for such behavior; a long-standing incapacity to develop emotional attachments; high or low intelligence that can thwart the therapeutic process; and the clinician's intense countertransference fear for his or her personal safety. In short, the more the patient resembles the dynamic profile of the pure psychopath, the less likely the patient is to respond to dynamic psychotherapy.

Antisocial patients with narcissistic features may be somewhat more amenable to psychotherapy. They may reveal some dependency in the transferences, and their internal "ideal object" may be somewhat less aggressive than in the pure psychopath (Meloy, 1988). The presence of major depression may reflect amenability to psychotherapy (Woody, McLellan, Lubovsky, & O'Brien, 1985). Turkat (1990) notes that the "hurting sociopath" who is sincerely and genuinely distressed has the potential to profit from psychotherapy. However, the most important predictor of treatment success is the ability to form a therapeutic alliance. Gertsley and colleagues (1989) showed a significant association between the ability to form a therapeutic alliance and treatment outcome in their study of 48 methadone-maintained male opiate addicts who met the criteria for antisocial personality disorder.

Parenthetically, a study of sex difference in treatment recommendations for antisocial personality is thought provoking. A survey was undertaken involving 119 clinical psychologists who responded to case histories depicting either a man or a woman with antisocial personality disorder and somatization. Results showed that clinicians were less likely to diagnose antisocial personality disorder correctly for female than for male patients. Women were consistently given better prognoses and were more likely to be recommended for insight-oriented psychotherapy than were men, who were given poorer prognoses and were more likely to be recommended for group therapy and legal constraints (Fernbach, Winstead, & Derlega, 1989).

Therapeutic stance and intervention strategy and techniques are other important factors in the treatment outcome equation. The traditional dynamic stance of neutrality is contraindicated. Gabbard (1994) contends that neutrality is tantamount to silent endorsement of or collusion with the antisocial patient's actions. Instead, the recommended therapeutic stance is active and confrontative. The clinician will need repeatedly to confront the patient's minimization and denial of antisocial behavior. Furthermore, confrontation must focus on here-and-now behavior rather than on analysis of unconscious material from the past.

From a dynamic perspective, it is crucial for the clinician to assist the patient in linking actions with internal states. Finally, the clinician's expectation for therapeutic change must be starkly realistic. Gabbard (1994) cautions that antisocial patients take delight in thwarting the clinician's wishes for them to change.

Countertransference issues are important in working with antisocial patients. Two common forms are disbelief and collusion (Symington, 1980). Disbelief involves the clinician's rationalization that the patient is not really "that bad." Collusion is perhaps the most problematic type of countertransference. Gabbard insists that the clinician be stable, persistent, and thoroughly incorruptible, as these patients will do whatever is necessary to corrupt the clinician into dishonest or unethical behavior. Through simulated tearfulness, sadness, or remorse, they can manipulate the clinician into empathizing with them.

As noted previously, there are studies of dynamic treatment with antisocial patients. One study of severe personality disordered individuals, including those with antisocial personality-disorder, found that significant split self-representations were present in the 27 patients studied. Relaxation exercises and a merging intervention were utilized to reduce the amnestic barriers that maintained this compartmentalization. Results showed that 24 of the patients responded with reduced resistance, increased treatment compliance, and improved daily functioning (Glantz & Goisman, 1990).

COGNITIVE-BEHAVIORAL APPROACH

Beck et al. (1990) provide an extended discussion of the cognitive therapy approach to persons with an antisocial personality disorder. They note that it is particularly difficult to develop a collaborative working relationship with these patients, who are likely to distrust the therapist, are uncomfortable with accepting help, and have little motivation because of the therapist's countertransference. Establishing rapport requires the therapist to avoid, or disengage from, positions of control or power struggles with such patients, as well as to admit vulnerability to their manipulativeness. Since these individuals are likely to lie, the therapist can avoid entrapment in the role of being the arbiter of the truth by admitting that it could happen. To avoid premature termination, it is suggested that the therapist work gradually to establish trust, explicitly acknowledge the antisocial individual's strengths and capabilities, and refrain from pressing the individual to acknowledge weaknesses. Premature termination also may occur if the individual's distress (i.e., depression or anxiety symptoms) is quickly alleviated. In such instances, Beck et al. suggest pointing out that continuing in therapy is in the patient's best interest and identifying any remaining distress that he or she may be denying or minimizing.

After treatment goals have been agreed upon, focusing on specific problem situations with problem-solving and behavioral strategies is suggested. If there is lack of impulse control, or acting out, or inappropriate expressions of anger, impulse-control and anger-management strategies are advised. As these individuals become better able to control their impulses and to anticipate the consequences of their actions, shifting the therapeutic focus to automatic thoughts and underlying schemas is possible. This transition from a largely behavioral focus to a more cognitive one gradually allows these individuals to become less vulnerable and more comfortable with disclosing their thoughts and feelings. As planned termination of treatment approaches, the focus shifts to the social pressures the person faces to continue antisocial behavior. Relapse-prevention strategies are useful in sensitizing these patients to people, places, and circumstances that are potential triggers for antisocial thinking and behaviors. Presuming that the individual has learned sufficient social skills to fit into prosocial groups, the likelihood of effective coping in the face of social pressures is increased. Beck et al. note that group and family therapy can be a useful adjunct to individual treatment.

Finally, Freeman, Pretzer, Simon, and Fleming (1990) believe that cognitive therapy can be effective not only in reducing antisocial behavior, but also in assisting the individual to adopt a more prosocial lifestyle. They caution that these patients often terminate treatment prematurely, unless they experience sufficient distress from an Axis I condition that provides an incentive for continuing to work in treatment.

Interpersonal Approach

For Benjamin (1993), psychotherapeutic interventions with persons with antisocial personality disorders can be planned and evaluated in terms of whether they enhance collaboration, facilitate learning about maladaptive patterns and their roots, block these patterns, enhance the will to change, and effectively encourage new patterns.

Benjamin notes that antisocial individuals do not respond well to individual psychotherapy alone. However, when combined with other modalities, such as milieu therapy, a positive treatment outcome may be possible. The goal of the collaborative phase of treatment is to establish a bonding and some degree of interdependence. Since collaboration in individual psychotherapy cannot be coerced and is seldom chosen by antisocial individuals, Benjamin suggests joining the individual in his or her initial hostile position, and then progressing toward collaboration. Other ways of eliciting collaboration suggested are utilizing sports heroes as role models or allowing the antisocial individual to assume a teaching role in supervised, socially acceptable settings. Wilderness survival training is another potential modality. In these instances, nurturance and bonding could be facilitated. Carefully managed group therapy can provide opportunities for bonding and control.

Once bonding and interdependence begin, the preconditions for collaboration have been met. Next, the antisocial individual is helped to recognize and understand the self-destructive features of the exploitive lifestyle and pattern. Benjamin believes that these individuals can then begin to develop the necessary self-management and social skills, such as self-care, delay of gratification, and empathy for others. However, she offers little discussion and few suggestions for facilitating change for individuals with this disorder.

GROUP THERAPY

Structured forms of group therapy may be quite effective with patients with antisocial personality disorders. As open, exploratory, and nondirective groups (Yalom, 1985) with heterogeneous compositions are easily disrupted by antisocial patients, such groups are not advisable (Liebowitz, Stone, & Turkat, 1986).

Three types of group treatment have been utilized with this type of patient: psychoeducational, psychotherapy, and support (Walker, 1992). Psychoeducational groups often didactic presentations by the clinician, which are then processed by the group members. Content and agenda are structured, as is patient participation. The group is composed of antisocial patients who meet given criteria for participation, and are chosen by the clinician. The groups are time limited and meet weekly for 90-minute sessions. Because of the complexity of these patients' interpersonal and other problems, these groups have limited utility for antisocial patients.

Psychotherapy groups have somewhat less structure than do psychoeducational groups, but make use of cohesive themes relevant to these patients. Group membership is determined by the clinician, who is in charge of both content and process. These groups tend to be long term, to meet weekly for 90 minutes, and are limited to nine or 10 patients. Because a group of 10 antisocial patients can be quite formidable, two clinician group therapists are recommended.

Two group therapists serve to diminish the group's potential for acting out against the group leaders, as one clinician is an easy target for isolation, as well as for attack or dismissal by group members. Two group leaders also offer patients more opportunity for constructive identification because of differences in the clinicians' personalities and styles. Furthermore, this coleadership allows for a "good guy/bad guy" routine, and permits "lateral passes" by the leaders, who may find themselves unable to handle a particular issue or patient (Walker, 1992).

Support groups are useful for antisocial patients who have had intensive inpatient or outpatient group psychotherapy. Although they are based on a self-help model, they are led by a clinician. The main focus of these ongoing groups with open membership is relapse prevention and the development of peer support.

Walker (1992) describes some useful guidelines for setting up these three different types of groups, as well as a number of rules and specific procedures for doing group work with antisocial patients.

MARITAL AND FAMILY THERAPY

A considerable number of studies have been published on the family dynamics and treatment of the antisocial patient, most of which relate to delinquent youths (Glueck & Glueck, 1950; Minuchin et al., 1976). A few studies suggest that short-term family therapy can also be effective with delinquent adolescents (Alexander & Parsons, 1973; Parsons & Alexander, 1973). Harbir (1981) notes that antisocial patients are seldom motivated to engage in family therapy, but to the extent that the clinician is able to engage the patient's parents or spouse, the more likely is the possibility of therapeutic change. As the antisocial patient tends to leave outpatient treatment precipitously when difficult and anxiety-provoking issues are faced, it is incumbent on the clinician to maximize therapeutic leverage. Specifically, this means establishing a consistent therapeutic alliance and involving the family at the outset, usually at the beginning of hospital treatment, as part of a court stipulation or as a required adjunct to residential treatment.

A major treatment goal is to help family members, or the spouse in couples therapy, to set limits on the patient. Typically, family members and spouses have minimized, ignored, or acted inconsistently in the face of the patient's antisocial behavior. As the family or spouse consistently sets and enforces limits, the patient's pathological behavior is reduced, and sometimes treatment-amenable symptoms, such as depression, emerge. This suggests that the patient is beginning to change and is more motivated to stop destructive behaviors. As family treatment proceeds, changes in destructive communication patterns can be achieved systematically (Parsons & Alexander, 1973).

MEDICATION

Few pharmacological investigations of the antisocial personality disorder per se have been reported. Kellner (1978, 1981, 1986) and Reid and Burke (1989) offer rather complete reviews of the use of various classes of psychotropics in the treatment of antisocial personality disorders.

Essentially, clinical research findings indicate that various benzodiazepines and antipsychotics have had limited efficacy or produced inconsistent results. There was considerable optimism that stimulants such as methylphenidate (Ritalin) or pemoline would be effective with antisocial patients with symptoms of attention-deficit disorder (Satterfield & Contwell, 1975), but there have been no controlled studies to support their use. Maintenance therapy with lithium carbonate also holds some promise for managing individuals with impulsive, violent explosive traits or mood swings (Sheard, 1976). However, many antisocial patients cannot tolerate its side effects or comply with treatment instructions and regimens. Nevertheless, patients with a positive family history of lithium-responsive illness, recurrent depression, or aggression are very good candidates for a lithium trial (Liebowitz, Stone, & Turkat, 1986). Beta-blockers such as propranolol also have been utilized for their antiaggressive effects (Yudofsky, William, & Gorman, 1981; Ratey, Morrill, & Oxenburg, 1983).

Evidence that altering serotonergic activity in the brain with selective serotonin reuptake inhibitors can reduce impulsive behavior has been published. At least four open trials have reported the efficacy of fluoxetine (Prozac) in patients with antisocial personality disorder (Coccaro, 1993). Kavoussi, Liu, and Coccaro (1994) reported in an open trial study that sertraline (Zoloft) is also effective with aggressiveness and impulsivity.

COMBINED AND INTEGRATED TREATMENT APPROACHES

Despite widespread pessimism about the treatability of this disorder, there is reason for cautious optimism provided that treatment is combined or multimodal and tailored to the particular needs and circumstances of the individual. There is clear evidence that time itself is the most effective treatment modality. In other words, the intensity of antisocial behaviors tends to dissipate with age (Regier, Boyd, Burke, et al., 1988). Purportedly that is the result of the cumulative effects of personal, social, legal, and financial repercussions of antisocial behavior. The next most effective treatment is specialized treatment—therapeutic communities or wilderness programs that provide firm limits and structure, group work with peers, and a structured work program (Woody et al., 1985). To the extent that sufficient therapeutic leverage is present in outpatient settings, treatment outcomes for antisocial patients can be at least guardedly optimistic.

As with borderline personality disorder, most agree that pharmacotherapy should not be the only treatment for antisocial personality disorder (Gunderson, 1986). Kellner (1986) suggests that treatment often begins with a psychotherapeutic modality, after which a trial of medication may be considered for a specific target symptom such as impulsivity, aggressiveness, explosiveness, or violence. In many instances, treatment will be long because of the patient's unwillingness or inability to persevere. Or it may consist of a few sessions interspersed with long intervals without any therapeutic work or for medication monitoring only. In any case, the clinician must attempt to establish a therapeutic alliance while maintaining firm limits. Psychoeducation, whether in an individual or group format, is usually necessary. Kellner (1986) notes that data support the use of sustained treatment, which invariably involves psychotherapies—individual, group, and family; behavior therapy; and psychoeducation—aimed at teaching self-control and postponement of gratification, as well as the use of medication. Although such interventions are exceedingly complex and difficult to implement, Kellner believes that they can make a substantial difference in the lives and adjustments of these patients.

CHAPTER 3

Avoidant Personality Disorder

The avoidant personality disorder found its way into DSM-III amid considerable controversy, with some contending that there was little distinction between the avoidant personality disorder and the schizoid and dependent personality disorders (Gunderson, 1983). However, the criteria in DSM-IV have been modified to differentiate the three sufficiently. Essentially, avoidant patients long for close interpersonal relationships, but fear humiliation, rejection, and embarrassment, and so avoid and distance themselves from others. Schizoid patients have little or no desire for close interpersonal relationships, which accounts for their distancing and avoidance of others. Similarly, while those with dependent personality disorders may be timid, submissive, and clinging because of their excessive need for attachment, persons with avoidant personality disorders are characterized by a fear of humiliation and rejection that results in social timidity and withdrawal.

This disorder has a relatively low prevalence in the general population that is estimated to be between 0.5 and 1.0 percent. In clinical settings, the disorder has been noted in approximately 10 percent of outpatients.

This chapter describes the characteristic features of the avoidant personality disorder and its related personality style, five different clinical formulations, psychological assessment indicators, and a variety of treatment approaches and intervention strategies.

CHARACTERISTICS OF THE AVOIDANT PERSONALITY STYLE AND DISORDER

The avoidant personality can be thought of as spanning a continuum from healthy to pathological, with the avoidant personality style at the healthy end and the avoidant personality disorder at the pathological end. Table 3.1 compares and contrasts differences between the avoidant style and disorder.

Table 3.1
A Comparison of Avoidant Personality Style Versus Disorder

Personality Style	*Personality Disorder*
• Comfortable with habit, repetition, and routine. Prefer the known to the unknown.	• Exaggerate the potential difficulties, physical dangers, or risks involved in doing something ordinary, but outside their usual routines.
• Close allegiance to family and/or a few close friends; tend to be homebodies.	• Have no close friends or confidants—or only one—other than first-degree relatives; avoid activities that involve significant interpersonal contact.
• Sensitive and concerned about what other think of them. Tend to be self-conscious and worriers.	• Unwilling to become involved with people unless certain of being liked; easily hurt by criticism or disapproval.
• Very discreet and deliberate in dealing with others.	• Fear being embarrassed by blushing, crying, or showing signs of anxiety in front of other people.
• Tend to maintain a reserved, self-restrained demeanor around others.	• Reticent in social situations because of a fear of saying something inappropriate or foolish, or of being unable to answer a question.
• Tend to be curious and can focus considerable attention on hobbies and avocations; however, a few engage in counterphobic coping behaviors.	• Tend to be underachievers, and find it difficult to focus on job tasks or hobbies.

The avoidant personality disorder is recognized by the following behavioral and interpersonal style, thinking or cognitive style, and emotional or affective style.

The behavioral style of avoidant personalities is characterized by social withdrawal, shyness, distrustfulness, and aloofness. Their behavior and speech are controlled, and they appear apprehensive and awkward. Interpersonally, they are sensitive to rejection. Even though they desire acceptance by others, they keep their distance and require unconditional approval before they are willing to "open up." They guardedly "test" others to determine who can be trusted to like them.

The cognitive style of avoidants can be described as perceptually vigilant; that is, they scan the environment looking for clues to potential threats or acceptance. Their thoughts are often distracted by their hypersensitivity. Not surprisingly, they have low self-esteem because of their devaluation of their achievements and their overemphasis on their own shortcomings.

Their affective or emotional style is marked by a shy and apprehensive quality. Because they are seldom able to obtain unconditional approval from others, they routinely experience sadness, loneliness, and tenseness. At times of increased distress, they will describe feelings of emptiness and depersonalization.

The following two case examples illustrate the differences between the avoidant personality style (Dr. Q.) and the avoidant personality disorder (Ms. A.).

Case Study: Avoidant Personality Disorder

Ms. A. is a 27-year-old student who contacted the University Counseling Center for help with "difficulty in concentrating." She indicated that the problem had started when her roommate of two years precipitously moved out to live with a boyfriend. Ms. A. described herself as being "blown away and hurt" by this. She noted that she had no close friends, and described herself as shy and as having had only one date since high school. Since then she had refused attempts by men to date her because of a previous rejection by a man who had dated her for a month and then never contacted her again. On examination, she had poor eye contact with the admissions counselor and appeared very shy and self-conscious.

Case Study: Avoidant Personality Style

Peter Q. is a 31-year-old eye surgeon who had recently been hired by a large HMO hospital and clinic after completing his residency training. Being new, attractive, and single, he was quickly noticed by the female staff.

His specialty was cataracts and laser surgery, at which he was exquisitely skilled, and he was respected by his patients. Although courteous, he was somewhat distant and shy emotionally. Dr. Q. seldom participated in staff gatherings, and if he did make an appearance, he would politely excuse himself when his beeper sounded—which seemed to be constantly—and he would not return. His social life seemed to be a mystery, and he had little contact with his male colleagues after hours, except for one. Dr. S. had run into Peter at a Civil War convention in another city, where he learned of Peter's long-standing hobby and collection of Civil War books and memorabilia. The two eventually became very good friends, spending considerable time together. Dr. S. recalls Peter's saying how he often daydreamed about being a Confederate general leading his troops to victory. Although he had his own apartment, Peter spent much of his free time at home with his parents. Dr. S. soon became a regular guest at the Q. home, and was surprised at how warm, cordial, and comfortable Peter was in this small setting as compared with the hospital.

DSM-IV Description and Criteria

Avoidant personalities seemingly are shy, lonely, and hypersensitive, and have low self-esteem. Although they are desperate for interpersonal involvement, they avoid contact with others because of their fear of social disapproval and rejection. In this regard, they are quite different from the schizoid personality, who has little, if any, interest in personal contact. Table 3.2 presents the description and criteria for this disorder according to DSM-IV.

FORMULATIONS OF THE AVOIDANT PERSONALITY DISORDER

Psychodynamic Formulation

Shyness, shame, and avoidant behaviors are conceptualized as defenses against embarrassment, humiliation, rejection, and failure (Gabbard, 1990). Shame and fear of exposure of the self to others are interconnected. Individuals with avoidant personalities tend to feel ashamed of their self-perceptions as weak, unable to compete, physically or mentally defective, or disgusting and unable to control bodily functions (Wurmser, 1981). Shame evolves from many different developmental experiences throughout the early childhood years. These developmental experiences, plus a constitutional predisposition to avoid stressful situations, tend to be reactivated in the avoidant patient upon exposure to individuals who matter a great deal to the patient (Gabbard, 1994).

Table 3.2
DSM-IV Criteria for Avoidant Personality Disorder*

301.82 Avoidant Personality Disorder

A pervasive pattern of social inhibition, feelings of inadequacy, and hypersensitivity to negative evaluation, beginning by early adulthood and present in a variety of contexts, as indicated by four (or more) of the following:

(1) avoids occupational activities that involve significant interpersonal contact, because of fears of criticism, disapproval, or rejection

(2) is unwilling to get involved with people unless certain of being liked

(3) shows restraint within intimate relationships because of the fear of being shamed or ridiculed

(4) is preoccupied with being criticized or rejected in social situations

(5) is inhibited in new interpersonal situations because of feelings of inadequacy

(6) views self as socially inept, personally unappealing, or inferior to others

(7) is unusually reluctant to take personal risks or to engage in any new activities because they may prove embarrassing

*Reprinted with permission from the *Diagnostic and Statistical Manual of Mental Disorders, Fourth Edition.* Copyright 1994 American Psychiatric Association.

Biosocial Formulation

Millon (1981) and Millon and Everly (1985) believe that the etiology and development of this personality disorder represent an interactive constellation of biogenical environmental factors. They hypothesize that the vigilance characterizing this personality reflects functional dominance of the sympathetic nervous system with a lowered autonomic arousal threshold. This could allow irrelevant impulses to intrude on logical association and diminish control and direction of thought and memory processes, resulting in a marked interface with normal cognitive processes. Research cited by Kagan, Reznick, and Snidman (1988) suggests that the trait of shyness is of genetic-constitutional origin, which requires specific environmental experiences to develop into a full-blown pattern of timidity and avoidance.

Parental and peer group rejection are two critical and prevalent environmental influences. The amount of parental rejection appears to be particularly intense and/or frequent. When peer group rejection reinforces parental rejection, the child's sense of self-worth and self-competence tend to be severely eroded, and result in self-critical attitudes. As a result, these individuals restrict their social experiences, are hypersensitive to rejection, and become excessively introspective. By restricting their social environment, they fail to develop social competence, which tends to evoke the ridicule of others for their asocial behavior. Because of their hypersensitivity and hypervigilence, they are prone to interpret minor rebuffs as principal indicators of rejection, where no rejection was intended. Finally, because of their excessive introspection, they are forced to examine the painful conditions they have created for themselves. Not surprisingly, they conclude that they do not deserve to be accepted by others.

Cognitive-Behavioral Formulation

According to Beck et al. (1990), individuals with avoidant personalities are fearful of initiating relationships, as well as of responding to others' attempts to relate to them because of their overriding belief that they will be rejected. For them, such rejection is unbearable, and so they engage in social avoidance. Furthermore, they engage in cognitive and emotional avoidance by not thinking about things that could cause them to feel dysphoric. Because of their low tolerance for dysphoria, they further distract themselves from their negative cognitions. Underlying these avoidance patterns are maladaptive schemas or long-standing dysfunctional beliefs about self and others. Schemas about self include themes of being different, inadequate, defective, and unlikable. Schemas about others involve themes of uncaring and rejection.

These individuals are likely to predict and interpret the rejection as caused solely by their personal deficiencies. This prediction of rejection results in dysphoria. Finally, avoidant individuals do not have internal criteria by which to judge themselves in a positive manner. Thus they must rely on their perceptions. They tend to misread a neutral or positive reaction as negative, which further compounds their rejection sensitivity and social, emotional, and cognitive avoidance. In short, they hold negative schemas that lead them to avoid situations where they could interact with others. They also avoid tasks that could engender uncomfortable feelings, and avoid thinking about matters that produce dysphoria. Because of their low tolerance for discomfort, they utilize distractions, excuse making, and rationalizations when they begin to feel sad or anxious.

Turkat (1990) describes this disorder as primarily anxiety based, and as characterized by timidity and anxiety concerning evaluation, rejection, and humiliation. He notes that the disorder is very responsive to behavioral interventions, particularly anxiety management desensitization methods, where the hierarchy is based on fear of rejection, criticism, or evaluation.

Interpersonal Formulation

According to Benjamin (1993), persons diagnosed with avoidant personality disorders tended to begin their developmental sequence with appropriate nurturance and social bonding. As a result, they continued to desire social contact and nurturance, but were subjected to relentless parental control with regard to creating an impressive social image. Visible flaws were a cause for great embarrassment and humiliation, particularly for the family. Besides exhortations to be admirable, they experienced degrading mockery for failures, personal imperfections, or shortcomings. The adult consequence is that avoidant individuals are socialized to perform adequately and manage an appropriate impression while avoiding occasions for embarrassment or humiliation. Typically, this humiliation was associated with exclusion, banishment, or rejection. As a result, they anticipate rejection and thus isolate themselves socially. Because they are well bonded, they crave relationships and social contacts, but must be convinced that there will be little or no risk of rejection or dejection.

Furthermore, although they experienced rejection and ridicule from their families, they also internalized the belief that the family is their source of support. Thus they have intense family loyalty, while harboring equally intense fears of outsiders. In short, avoidant individuals exhibit an intense fear of humiliation and rejection. To avoid this, they socially withdraw and restrain themselves, while praying for love and acceptance. They can become very intimate with a select few who pass their highly stringent safety test. Occasionally, they can lose control and explode with rageful indignation.

Integrative Formulation

The following integrative formulation may be helpful in understanding how the avoidant personality disorder is likely to have developed.

Biologically, the avoidant personality was likely to have been a hyperirritable and fearful infant. In Thomas and Chess's classification (1977), the avoidant would likely have exhibited the "slow-to-warm-up" infant temperament. Millon and Everly (1985) suggest that avoidant personalities often experienced maturational irregularities as children. This, as well as a hyperirritable pattern, is attributable in part to a low arousal threshold of the autonomic nervous system.

Psychologically, avoidants view themselves, others, the world, and life's purpose in terms of the following themes. They tend to view themselves by some variant of the theme: "I'm inadequate and frightened of rejection." They see themselves as chronically tense, fatigued, and self-conscious, and they devalue their achievements by their self-critical attitude. They tend to see the world as some variant of the theme: "Life is unfair—people reject and criticize me—but I still want someone to like me." As such, they are likely to conclude: "Therefore, be vigilant, demand reassurance, and if all else fails, fantasize and daydream about the way life could be." The most common defense mechanism of the avoidant personality is fantasy.

Socially, predictable patterns of parenting and environmental factors can be noted for the avoidant personality disorder. The avoidant personality is likely to have experienced parental rejection or ridicule. Later, siblings and peers are likely to continue this pattern of rejection and ridicule. The parental injunction is likely to have been, "We don't accept you, and probably no one else will either." They may have had parents with high standards, and worried that they may not have or would not meet these standards and so would not be accepted.

This avoidant pattern is confirmed, reinforced, and perpetuated by the following individual and systems factors: a sense of personal inadequacy

Table 3.3
Characteristics of Avoidant Personality Disorder

1.	Behavioral appearance	Shy, mistrustful, aloof; apprehensive, socially awkward; controlled, underactive behavior; feelings of emptiness and depersonalization
2.	Interpersonal behavior	Guardedly "tests" others; rejection sensitive as self-protectant; desires acceptance, but maintains distance; has interpersonal skills, but fears using them
3.	Cognitive style	Perpetual vigilance; thoughts easily distracted by hypersensitivity
4.	Feeling style	Shy and apprehensive
5.	Parental injunction/ environmental factors	"We don't accept you, and probably nobody else will either." Parental rejection and/or ridicule; later, peer group alienation
6.	Biological/temperament	Hyperirritable infantile pattern; low arousal threshold for autonomic nervous system
7.	Self view	"I'm inadequate and frightened of rejection." Chronically tense, fatigued, self-conscious; devalue own achievements, self-critical
8.	World view	"Life is unfair, people reject and criticize me, but I want someone to like me. Therefore, be vigilant, demand reassurance, and, if all else fails, fantasize and daydream."
9.	Self and perpetuant	Fear of social rejection and humiliation, hypervigilance, restricted social experiences (+) catastrophizing→ increased hypervigilance and hypersensitivity, increased self-pity→ reinforcement of avoidant style

and a fear of rejection leading to hypervigilance, which leads to restricted social experiences. These experiences, plus catastrophic thinking, lead to increased hypervigilance and hypersensitivity, leading to self-pity, anxiety, and depression, which lead to further confirmation of avoidant beliefs and styles (Sperry & Mosak, 1993).

ASSESSMENT OF AVOIDANT PERSONALITY DISORDER

Several sources of information are useful in establishing a diagnosis and treatment plan for personality disorders. Observation, collateral information, and psychological testing are important adjuncts to the patient's self-report in the clinical interview. This section briefly describes some characteristic observations that the clinician makes and the nature of the rapport likely to develop in initial encounters with specific personality-disordered individuals. Characteristic response patterns on various objective (i.e., MMPI-2 and MCMI-II) and projective (i.e., Rorschach and TAT) tests are also described.

In the initial interview, these individuals tend to be monosyllabic, circumstantial, and guarded. Some may even appear suspicious or quite anxious, but all are hypersensitive to rejection and criticism. Reluctance and guardedness should be approached with empathy and reassurance. The clinician does well to avoid confrontation, which most likely will be interpreted as criticism. Instead, he or she should use empathic responses that encourage the sharing of past pain and anticipatory fears. When these individuals feel that the clinician understands their hypersensitivity and will be protective of them, they are willing to trust and cooperate with treatment. After they feel safe and accepted, the character of the interview can change dramatically. Rapport has been achieved, and they feel relieved when they can describe their fears of being embarrassed and criticized and their sensitivity to being misunderstood. They may experience these fears of being embarrassed as silly and express this. If the clinician identifies with the position, they are likely to feel ridiculed and to withdraw again (Othmer & Othmer, 1989).

The Minnesota Multiphasic Personality Inventory (MMPI-2), the Million Clinical Multiaxial Inventory (MCMI-II), the Rorschach Psychodiagnostic Test, and the Thematic Apperception Test (TAT) can be useful in diagnosing the avoidant personality disorder, as well as the avoidant personality style or trait.

On the MMPI-2, a 2–7/7–2 (Depression–Psychasthenia) profile is typical. This profile reflects depression about assumed rejection, as well as apprehension and self-doubt about relating to others. When social withdrawal is also present, a high score on O (Social Introversion) is likely, as well as a lower 9 (Hypomania) scale. When social withdrawal and self-rejection lead to decreased functioning, an elevation on scale 8 (Schizophrenia) may occur (Meyer, 1993).

On the MMCI-II, an elevation of 85 or above on scale 2 (Avoidant), along with low scores on 4 (Histrionic) and 7 (Obsessive-Compulsive), is likely. Moderate elevations on scales 8B (Self-defeating) and C (Borderline) may also be present. The higher S (Schizotypal) is elevated, the more likely it is that decompensation has occurred (Meyer, 1993).

On the Rorschach, blocked or relatively inactive M (Human Movement) responses are likely. A high number of P (Popular) responses occur, and C (Contrast) often involves passive animals such as deer and rabbits—sometimes being maimed or killed—or passive interactions in the M responses (Meyer, 1993).

TREATMENT APPROACHES AND INTERVENTIONS

Treatment Considerations

Included in a differential diagnosis of the avoidant personality disorder are other Axis II personality disorders: schizoid personality disorder, schizotypal personality disorder, borderline personality disorder, and dependent personality disorder. The most common Axis I syndromes associated with the avoidant personality disorder are agoraphobia, social phobia, generalized anxiety disorder, dysthymia, major depressive episode, hypochondriasis, conversion disorder, dissociative disorder, and schizophrenia. Recent investigations indicate that there are two subtypes of social phobia, "circumscribed" and "generalized" (Liebowitz, Stone, & Turkat, 1986). The traditional description of social phobia is the circumscribed subtype. The generalized type involves fear and avoidance of a wide range of social and performance situations. For instance, patients may be unable to attend social functions, return goods to a store, and the like. Considerable overlap exists between generalized social phobia and avoidant personality disorder. The treatment implications, particularly regarding pharmacotherapy, are described later in this chapter. It has been said that next to the borderline personality disorder, the avoidant personality disorder is the most labile and likely to decompensate (Reid, 1989).

In terms of treatment goals and strategies, there are relatively few clinical case reports and almost no controlled research on treating the avoidant personality. Nevertheless, Frances and Clarkin (1981) believe that those with avoidant personality disorders are excellent candidates for various psychotherapeutic approaches, with the choice depending on the patient's goals, preferences, and psychological mindedness, and the clinician's expertise. Generally, the goal of therapy should be to increase the individual's self-esteem and confidence in relationship to others, and to desensitize the individual to the criticism of others. Finally, irrespective of the type of treatment approach, it is useful to note that avoidant personalities tend to evoke two types of countertransference—therapeutic protectiveness or excessive overambitiousness—in clinicians. In the first instance, the clinician insulates patients from risk, thus reaffirming their self views of insecurity and weakness. In the second instance, the patients are forced to face new situations prematurely without adequate preparation, and are then criticized for failing to be braver.

INDIVIDUAL PSYCHOTHERAPIES

Psychodynamic Psychotherapy

Both expressive and supportive aspects of psychodynamic psychotherapy can be most effective in treating avoidant personality disorders (Gabbard, 1994). The supportive aspect involves an empathic appreciation of the humiliation and embarrassment associated with exposure to fearful interpersonal circumstances and the pain connected with rejection. It also involves the clinician's prescription of exposure to the feared situation. Firm encouragement, of course, must accompany this prescription. More of their fantasies and anxieties will be activated in the actual situation of exposure than in their defensive posture of withdrawal. Explaining this fact will further encourage avoidant patients to seek out fearful situations.

The expressive aspect of therapy focuses on exploring the underlying causes of shame as related to past developmental experiences. To the extent that the patient is willing to risk confronting the feared circumstance, the expressive aspect of therapy is greatly enhanced. Initial exploratory efforts can be frustrating in that avoidant individuals may be somewhat uncertain about whom it is they fear. They tend to provide vague and global explanations such as "rejection" and "shyness" rather than specific fantasies. Thus the clinician does well to explore specific fantasies within the context of the transference.

These individuals tend to have a considerable degree of anxiety about the psychotherapeutic requirement to share thoughts and feelings openly. Accordingly, when they react nonverbally (such as blush) to something that has been verbalized, the clinician might ask them to share their embarrassment and what they imagine the clinician could be thinking and feeling. By pursuing the details of specific situations, these patients can develop a greater awareness of the correlates of the shame affect (Gabbard, 1994).

Interpretive techniques are also useful either as the primary intervention or as adjunctive to behavioral and interpersonal approaches. The basic strategy involves interpretive unconscious fantasies that their fear or impulses will become uncontrollable and harmful to self and others. Not surprisingly, their avoidant behavior maintains a denial of unconscious wishes or impulses (Mackinnon & Michels, 1971). Furthermore, these patients tend to have harsh superegos and subsequently project their own unrealistic expectations of themselves onto others. In so doing, they evade expected criticism and embarrassment by avoiding relationships with others. A complete interpretation identifies the unconscious impulse and the fear, and traces the resulting avoidant defensive pattern in early life experiences, in outside relationships, and in the transference (Fenichel, 1945).

Cognitive-Behavioral Approach

Beck et al. (1990) provide an in-depth discussion of the cognitive therapy approach with avoidant personalities. These individuals are often difficult to engage in treatment, given their basic strategy of avoidance and their hypersensitivity to perceived criticism. The therapist must work diligently, yet carefully, at building trust. Trust tests are common in the early stage of treatment, and can include a pattern of canceling appointments or having difficulty scheduling regular appointments. It is important not to challenge automatic thoughts prematurely, as such challenges can be viewed as personal criticism. Only after these individuals are solidly engaged in treatment should the therapist use cognitive interactions to test their expectancies in social situations. To the extent that the therapist utilizes collaboration rather than confrontation and guided discovery rather than direct disputation, these individuals are more likely to view therapy as constructive and to remain in treatment.

Since they often experience high levels of interpersonal anxiety, it is useful to employ anxiety management interventions early in treatment. Because these individuals work at avoiding not only unpleasant affects, but also thinking about matters that elicit unpleasant feelings, it is useful to work in increasing emotional tolerance with desensitization methods and reframing. Furthermore, since they may not have learned the basics of social interaction, structured social skills training may need to be incorporated.

Later in therapy, when these individuals have achieved some of their short-term treatment goals and developed sufficient trust in the therapist, efforts to challenge automatic thoughts and to restructure maladaptive schemas are appropriate. Issues involving the risk of developing close relationships and intimacy are central. Typically, it is necessary to decatastrophize disapproval and rejection. To the extent that they have developed sufficient self-efficacy and have experienced enough success on a variety of levels of relationships, they are more receptive to entertaining the notion that disapproval in a close relationship does not equal rejection or devastation. Group therapy has a place in the treatment of this disorder, so that they can learn new attitudes and practice new skills in a socially benign and accepting environment. In summary, the cognitive therapy approach to this disorder recognizes the significant challenge of engaging the avoidant individual in treatment and utilizes efforts to build trust and reduce social anxiety and cognitive and emotional avoidance. It then proceeds to correcting social skills deficits with behavioral methods before turning to cognitive analysis and disputation of automatic thoughts and schemas, and provides a safe environment in which to try out socially proactive behavior.

From a behavioral perspective, management of the avoidant pattern is relatively straightforward (Turkat, 1990). Anxiety-management procedures, assertiveness and social skills training through role playing, direct instruction, and modeling are effective in developing confident social behavior. However, graded exposure is the most effective behavioral intervention strategy for extinguishing avoidant behavior and anxiety intolerance (Greist & Jefferson, 1992).

Paradoxical intention may prove useful, particularly with avoidant patients who are also oppositional. With this strategy, the patient seeks rejection in a way that is both predictable and under the patient's control. For instance, a single man with a fear of dating agrees to an experiment requiring that he be rejected for dates by two women in the coming week. If one of the women approached accepts his offer, he can go out with her, on the condition that he had asked out an additional woman, who had rejected him. In other words, being rejected becomes a treatment goal. This intervention reduces rejection sensitivity. Use of such a paradoxical intervention may work with the oppositionally avoidant patient by accentuating the patient's need to defeat the clinician by doing the opposite of what is suggested or prescribed (Weeks & L'Abate, 1982; Haley, 1978).

Interpersonal Approach

For Benjamin (1993), psychotherapeutic interventions with persons with avoidant personality disorders can be planned and evaluated in terms of whether they enhance collaboration, facilitate learning about maladaptive patterns and their roots, block these patterns, enhance the will to change, and effectively encourage new patterns.

Avoidant individuals already know how to relate to a select few individuals, and thus a supportive therapist can easily provide a safe haven for them. They respond favorably to accurate empathy and warm support. Gradually, as they share intimacies and feelings of inadequacy, guilt, or shame, they begin to increase self-acceptance. Only then can they realistically begin to explore maladaptive patterns. As they are exquisitely sensitive to criticism, premature confrontation must be avoided.

General reconstructive changes will occur only if these individuals understand and appreciate the impact of their maladaptive patterns in a way that helps them decide to change. Benjamin advocates couples therapy for avoidant patients in marriages or long-term relationships. Typically, these relationships are characterized by an intimacy that assures interpersonal distance and safety for the avoidant partner. Such a pattern of hiding on the margins of relationships is often rooted in unconscious loyalty to the family mandate that the avoidant individual remain isolated and safe. In couples therapy, the clinician would block attempts of partners to humiliate or trash each other that previously had justified the avoidant individual's withdrawal. The most difficult therapeutic task for avoidant individuals is deciding to sacrifice the benefits of their maladaptive patterns and accept the risk of developing new ones. Insight into their humiliation and their loyalty to abusive parents or siblings is insufficient. However, Benjamin believes that steady reassurance in a context of competent, protective instruction fosters this change. She advocates safe group therapy, wherein clinicians block "trashing" and critical appraisals, for helping avoidant individuals to accept themselves and to learn the basic relational skills they had missed learning earlier in life. This is not to say that training and other social skills cannot occur in individual therapy, but rather that they are greatly facilitated in a safe group context.

GROUP THERAPY

Patients with avoidant personality disorders typically fear group therapy in the same way that they fear other new and socially demanding situations. It is for this very reason that group therapy may be specifically and especially effective for avoidant patients who can be persuaded to undertake the exposure (Yalom, 1985). Empathetic group therapy can assist these individuals to overcome social anxieties and develop interpersonal trust and rapport.

A combination of cognitive therapy and social skills training appears to be effective. Alden (1989) included the following aspects of cognitive therapy in the group process: (1) identifying underlying fears, (2) becoming increasingly aware of the anxiety related to fears, and (3) shifting attentional focus from fear-related thinking to behavioral action. Didactic information, modeling, and the practice of role playing were basic techniques incorporated into the sessions. Stravynski, Grey, and Elie (1987) found that a briefer course of group therapy centered on social skills training can be highly effective in ameliorating social skills deficits that exacerbate anxiety about social relatedness.

These individuals tend to avoid activities that involve significant interpersonal contact for fear of being exposed or ridiculed. Therefore, it takes them longer to adapt to a group setting and to begin to participate actively in treatment. The group therapist's role in pacing the avoidant patient's disclosure and engagement within the group can be very important (Azima, 1983). Rennenberg, Goldstein, Phillips, et al. (1990) found clients with this disorder so extremely anxious and avoidant that proceeding directly to social skills training and behavioral rehearsal was unproductive. Stravynski et al. (1987) suggest beginning with progressive relaxation training and systematic desensitization. Behavioral reversal was used in the group for exposure, itself an effective treatment for social phobia (Stravynski, Marks, & Yule, 1982). Turner, Beidel, Dancu, et al. (1986) used communication and social skills training during behavioral rehearsal as well.

Structured activities will help avoidant individuals organize how they think and act so that they are more efficient in therapy. Alden (1989) established specific goals for patients to accomplish between sessions in order to enhance generalization from treatment sessions to daily life. The patients selected several social tasks to try, beginning with easy situations and progressing to more difficult ones. In the group setting, she also introduced interpersonal skills training. The process of friendship formation was presented, and clients were encouraged to incorporate these skills into their weekly social tasks. Four sets of behavioral skills that facilitate relating to others were described, modeled by therapists, and discussed and practiced by group members. These included listening/attending skills, empathic sensitivity, appropriate self-disclosure, and respectful assertiveness.

Rennenberg et al. (1990) found that treatment gains through group intervention were stable over one year, however, most patients continued with individual therapy after completing group treatment. It is quite possible that the continued therapy served to reinforce and maintain gains made during the group treatment program. Clinically important changes were reported by patients themselves or their individual therapists. Treated subjects reported decreases in their social reticence, less interference due to social anxiety at work and in social situations, fewer symptoms of social anxiety, and greater satisfaction with social activities (Alden, 1989).

MARITAL/FAMILY THERAPY

Although avoidant individuals need to recognize how their current dysfunctional patterns were developed, they also need to focus on their current interpersonal experiences with significant others in their lives. As patients with avoidant personality disorders generally provide clinicians with vague descriptions of their interpersonal experiences, others may be helpful in filling in important gaps in the information. Couples and family treatments may be indicated in order to establish a family structure that allows more room for interpersonal exploration outside the tightly closed family circle (Gurman & Kniskern, 1981). Benjamin (1993) advocates couples therapy for avoidant individuals in marriages or long-term relationships, as typically these are characterized by intimacy that assures interpersonal distance and safety for the avoidant partner.

MEDICATION

Until recently, most publications on the treatment of the avoidant personality have focused on psychotherapeutic interventions, and only a few studies of pharmacological treatment have been reported. The reluctance to view personality disorders as amenable to pharmacological treatment seems to account for the paucity of studies on the biological treatment of avoidant personality disorder (Deltito & Stam, 1989). Many of these patients fear medications and their side effects, just as they do any other new experience. Nevertheless, evidence is accumulating that some aspects of extreme social anxiety may be highly drug responsive. Recent data suggest that the avoidant personality disorder significantly overlaps with the global subtype of social phobia, also called generalized social phobia. This means that the use of monoamine oxidase inhibitors (MAOIs) or fluoxetine may prove quite useful for avoidant patients (Deltito & Stam, 1989). Liebowitz et al. (1986) also indicate that social phobia, in its generalized form, often overlaps with the avoidant personality disorder, and is quite responsive to MAOIs. Deltito and Perugi (1989) have documented a case of social phobia and avoidant personality disorder successfully treated with phenelzine. The patient showed improvement in specific fears of eating and speaking in public, as well as global improvements in terms of comfort, confidence, and assertiveness in social situations. In their studies, Liebowitz et al. (1986) administered phenelzine to a pure sample of patients with social phobias, with marked or moderate improvement for all subjects. The results demonstrated the disappearance of the physical manifestations of social anxiety, as well as increased comfort and initiative in work and social settings. A more recent study by Liebowitz, Schneier, Hollander, et al. (1991) has postulated that patients with discrete social phobias respond preferentially to beta-blockers whereas those with generalized social phobias respond best to MAOIs. A new generation of MAOIs is known by the acronym RIMA, for reversible inhibitors of monoamine oxidase A. Brofaromia and moclobemide are RIMAs that have proved effective in controlled studies . Unlike MAOIs, RIMAs do not require dietary restrictions. They remain investigational in the United States, however, and it may be a few years before the Food and Drug Administration approves them.

COMBINED/INTEGRATED TREATMENT APPROACH

Clinical experience reveals that many avoidant personalities are often unable to focus on the patient–clinician relationship to the extent necessary to work with a purely dynamic therapy. Similarly, many have difficulty with fully utilizing cognitive-behavioral interventions in the interpersonal context of therapy. Thus an integrative treatment strategy may be required. Alden (1992) describes an integration of the cognitive and the psychodynamic–interpersonal approaches. The cognitive is, of course, based on Beck and associates (1990) and the psychodynamic–interpersonal is based on the time-limited dynamic psychotherapy approach developed by Strupp and Binder (1984).

The cognitive-interpersonal patterns that characterize the avoidant personality are dysfunctional beliefs of being different or biologically defective, as well as beliefs that these defects and feelings are visible to others, who will react with disgust, disapproval, or dismissal. These individuals tend to protect themselves by looking to the clinician to provide direction, and by understating, or even withholding, feelings and reactions of which they fear the clinician will disapprove. Thus the clinician's primary task is to work collaboratively with patients to modify their cognitive–interpersonal style. Adler (1992) describes four steps in the integrative approach. The first step is recognition of treatment process issues. The clinician must quickly recognize that these patients tend to withhold or understate information that is clinically relevant. Clinicians should expect them to respond to direct questions with "I'm not sure" or "I don't know." Such evasive and avoidant responses characterize their thought processes and prevent them from encoding details about social encounters.

Clinicians may find themselves interpreting "resistance" or focusing on global and vague interpersonal beliefs and behavior as treatment targets. In either instance, both clinician and patient will experience discouragement and treatment outcomes will be limited. Furthermore, clinicians must recognize that avoidant patients' infectious "hopelessness" and depression are largely attributable to their inability to process positive information, their lack of attentiveness, and their firmly established negative beliefs and schemas.

The second step is increased awareness of cognitive–interpersonal patterns. Patients need to be encouraged to observe their interpersonal encounters outside of sessions by self-monitoring and keeping a diary. Adler notes four components of the interpersonal pattern: their beliefs and expectancy of other persons, the behavior that arises from these beliefs, others' reactions to them, and the conclusions they draw from the experiences. As this process of self-observation and analysis proceeds, these patients come to realize that their mutual understanding of their interpersonal problem is incomplete and a common pattern emerges. The clinician's role is to draw attention to the beliefs that underlie self-perception, which lead to self-protective behaviors.

The third step focuses on alternative strategies. As patients recognize and understand the cognitive–interpersonal pattern and style, the clinician can increase their motivation to try new behaviors by helping them recognize that their old and new views of self are in conflict, and that this conflict can be reconciled. Helping patients to integrate their current beliefs with their earlier interpersonal experiences helps them to understand that their social fears and expectations resulted in part from their temperament and parenting. As patients continue to identify and understand their cognitive–interpersonal patterns, they begin to try new strategies, either on their own or at the clinician's prompting.

The final step involves behavioral experimentation and cognitive evaluation. These therapeutic strategies are discussed in detail by Beck et al. (1990), to which the reader is referred. Friendship formation and assertive communication are the two basic interpersonal skills that avoidant patients must increase. Role playing and directed assignments are particularly useful in this regard. The section on social skills in Zimbardo (1977) has proved extremely useful as a handout for avoidant patients. Patients are gently guided through exercises to develop assertive communication skills. As a matter of fact, Zimbardo's entire book is an invaluable adjunct in the treatment of the avoidant personality.

Combined Treatment Approach

The basic premise of this book is that a single treatment modality such as psychotherapy may well be effective for the highest functioning personality-disordered individual, but will be less effective for moderate functioning and largely ineffective for more severely dysfunctional individuals. These lower functioning patients tend to be more responsive to combined treatment modalities, including integrative psychotherapeutic intervention with medication and group treatment such as group therapy or support groups. As noted in the discussion of group treatment, avoidant patients have considerable difficulty with any kind of group. Ideally, lower functioning avoidant patients should be involved in both individual and group therapy concurrently. When this is not possible, time-limited, skill-oriented group training sessions or a support group may be sufficient. As such patients' patterns of avoidance and social inhibition make entry into and continuation with therapeutic groups distressing, individual sessions should be focused on transitioning them into the group.

Medication is often necessary in the early stages of treatment, and can be particularly useful in reducing distress and self-protective behavior during the transition into concurrent group treatment.

CHAPTER 4

Borderline Personality Disorder

The borderline personality disorder has captured the attention of the mental health community as has no other diagnostic entity. Not only are increasing numbers of patients with borderline personality disorders showing up in the caseloads of mental health clinicians, but many clinicians are convinced that they are largely untreatable. The borderline personality disorder has been dubbed one of the most prevalent neurotic personalities of our times (Sperry, 1991a), and more books, articles, and research studies on this disorder have been published in the past five years than on any other psychiatric disorder. Workshops, seminars, and the subject of borderline pathology are ever present.

Previously, the borderline personality was called pseudoneurotic schizophrenia, schizophrenic character, ambulatory schizophrenia, or latent schizophrenia. Efforts to understand this condition, which seemed to be between or on the border of neurosis and psychosis, have occupied many psychoanalytic theorists and researchers, and more recently, descriptive and phenomenological researchers. Largely because of the increasing interest in and literature on this disorder, the borderline personality disorder was added to DSM-III. Prior to that, borderline patients often were diagnosed in the DSM-II category of schizophrenia, latent type. Dissatisfaction with the failure of DSM-III and DSM-III-R to account for brief psychotic

53

Table 4.1
Comparison of the Borderline Personality Style and Disorder

Personality Style	*Personality Disorder*
• Tend to experience passionate, focused attachments in all relationships. Nothing in the relationship is taken lightly.	• Pattern of unstable and intense relationships noted by alternating between extremes of over idealization and devaluation.
• Emotionally active and reactive, they show their feelings and put their hearts into everything.	• Impulsive in at least two areas that are potentially self-damaging, e.g., spending, sex, substance abuse, shoplifting, reckless driving, binge eating, suicidal threats, gestures, or behavior.
• Tend to be uninhibited, spontaneous, fun loving, and undaunted by risk.	• Affective instability marked by shifts from baseline mood to depression, irritability, or anxiety, usually lasting a few hours and only rarely more than a few days.
• Tend to be creative, lively, busy, and engaging individuals. They show initiative and can stir others to activity.	• Inappropriate, intense anger or lack of control of anger, e.g., frequent displays of temper, constant anger, recurrent physical fights; chronic feelings of emptiness or boredom.
• Imaginative and curious, they are willing to experience and experiment with other roles, cultures, and value systems.	• Marked and persistent identity disturbance marked by uncertainty about at least two of the following: self-image, sexual orientation, long-term goals or career choice, type of friends desired, preferred values.
• Regularly tend to become deeply involved in a romantic relationship with one person.	• Frantic efforts to avoid real or imagined abandonment.

episodes prompted the inclusion of transient, stress-related paranoid ideation of severe dissociative symptoms as a criterion in DSM-IV.

There remains concern about the designation of borderline: Is it a specific personality disorder, or is it a dimension of personality or a personality organization (Kernberg, 1984) or a spectrum disorder (Meissner, 1988)? If the designation of borderline refers to a continuum, then all the personality disorders in clusters A and B could be considered borderline conditions.

Estimates are that approximately 2 percent of the general population meet the criteria for this disorder, and that about 10 percent of outpatients and 20 percent of psychiatric inpatients have the disorder. Finally, clinical populations with personality disorders meet the criteria for borderline personality disorder.

This chapter describes the characteristic features of this disorder and its related personality style. Five different clinical formulations and psychological assessment indicators are highlighted. Also described are a variety of treatment approaches, modalities, and intervention strategies.

CHARACTERISTICS OF THE BORDERLINE PERSONALITY STYLE AND DISORDER

The borderline personality is characterized by the following behavior and interpersonal, cognitive, and emotional styles.

Behaviorally, borderlines are characterized by physically self-damaging acts, such as suicidal gestures, self-mutilation, or the provocation of fights. Their social and occupational accomplishments are often less than their intelligence and ability warrant. Of all the personality disorders, these patients are most likely to exhibit irregularities of circadian rhythms, especially of the sleep–wake cycle. Thus chronic insomnia is a common complaint.

Interpersonally, borderlines are characterized by their paradoxical instability. That is, they fluctuate quickly between idealizing and clinging to another individual and devaluing and opposing that individual. They are exquisitively sensitive to rejection, and experience abandonment depression following the slightest of stressors. Millon (1981) considers separation anxiety a primary motivator of this personality disorder. These individuals develop interpersonal relationships rather quickly and intensely, and yet their social adaptiveness is superficial. They are extraordinarily intolerant of being alone, and they go to great lengths to seek out the company of others, whether in indiscriminate sexual affairs, late-night telephone calls to relatives and recent acquaintances, or late-night visits to hospital emergency rooms with a host of vague medical or psychiatric complaints.

Their cognitive style is described as inflexible and impulsive (Millon, 1981). Their inflexibility is characterized by rigid abstractions that easily lead to grandiose, idealized perceptions of others, not as real people, but as personifications of "all good" or "all bad." They reason by analogy from the past, and thus have difficulty in reasoning logically and learning from past experiences and relationships. Because they have an external locus of control, borderlines usually blame others when things go wrong. By accepting responsibility for their own incompetence, they believe they would feel even more powerless to change circumstances. Accordingly, their emotions fluctuate between hope and despair because they believe that external circumstances are well beyond their control (Shulman, 1982). Their cognitive style is also marked by impulsivity, and just as they vacillate between idealization and devaluation of others, their thoughts shift from one extreme to another: "I like people; no, I don't like them"; "Having goals is good; no, it's not"; "I need to get my life together; no, I can't, it's hopeless." The inflexibility and impulsivity complicate the process of identity formation. Their uncertainty about self-image, gender identity, goals, values, and career choices reflects this impulsive and flexible stance.

Gerald Adler (1985) suggests that borderlines have an underdeveloped evocative memory, so that they find it difficult to recall images and feeling states that could structure and soothe them in times of turmoil. Their inflexibility and impulsivity are further noted in their tendency toward "splitting." Splitting is the inability to synthesize contradictory qualities, such that the individual views others as all good or all bad and utilizes "projective identification," that is, attributes his or her own negative or dangerous feelings to others. Their cognitive style is further characterized by an inability to tolerate frustration. Finally, micropsychotic episodes can be noted when these individuals are under a great deal of stress. These are ill-defined, strange thought processes, especially noted in response to unstructured rather than structured situations, and may take the form of derealization, depersonalization, intense rage reactions, unusual reactions to drugs, and intense brief paranoid episodes. Because of their difficulty in focusing their attention and the subsequent loss of relevant data, borderlines also have a diminished capacity to process information.

The emotional style of individuals with this disorder is characterized by marked mood shifts from a normal or euthymic mood to a dysphoric mood. In addition, inappropriate and intense anger and rage may be easily triggered. At the other extreme are feelings of emptiness, a deep "void," or boredom.

The following case examples further illustrate the differences between the borderline personality disorder (Mr. J.) and the borderline personality style (Janice P.).

Case Study: Borderline Personality Disorder

Mr. J. is a 31-year-old unemployed man who was referred to the hospital emergency room by his therapist at a community mental health center after two days of sustained suicidal gestures. He appeared to function adequately until his senior year in high school, when he became preoccupied with transcendental meditation. He had considerable difficulty with concentrating during his first semester of college, and seemed to focus most of his energy on finding a spiritual guru. At times, massive anxiety and feelings of emptiness swept over him, which he found would suddenly vanish if he lightly cut his wrist enough to draw blood. He had been in treatment with his current therapist for 18 months, and had become increasingly hostile and demanding as a patient, whereas earlier he had been quite captivated by his therapist's empathy and intuitive sense. Lately, his life seemed to center on these twice-weekly therapy sessions. Mr. J.'s most recent suicidal thoughts followed the therapist's disclosure that he was moving out of the area.

Case Study: Borderline Personality Style

Janice P. is a 29-year-old graduate student in Oriental literature. She had completed her undergraduate degree at the university in business and management with honors, and had planned on starting her M.B.A. degree that fall. A summer tour of Japan and China dramatically changed her life. She fell in love with the Orient: the people, the food, the customs, the ambiance, but especially with a literature professor whom she met at a Tokyo university. She fell madly in love with him the first time she saw him at a chance meeting, and spent the two weeks before her flight back to the United States totally engrossed with his poetry, his stories, and his life. He was married, but his wife was away on a vacation. Janice was conflicted about returning home even though the professor had broken off the relationship. She entreated him to leave his wife, and was crushed that he would not do so. She returned to the university with an ardent desire to immerse herself in the study of Oriental literature. She had fantasies of going back to Tokyo as a visiting professor and working with the "love of her life," with the goal of eventually having him all to herself. Even though she was doing well in her classes, she occasionally got in touch with the anger and hurt she had experienced that summer. Midway through her first semester in graduate school, she met an Oriental graduate student, with whom she instantly fell in love.

DSM-IV Description and Criteria

Table 4.2 gives the DSM-IV description and criteria.

FORMULATIONS OF THE BORDERLINE PERSONALITY DISORDER

Psychodynamic Formulations

Kernberg (1975) targets the rapprochement subphase of Mahler's separation–individuation developmental theory as the point of fixation for bor-

Table 4.2.
DSM-IV Description and Criteria for Borderline Personality Disorder*

301.83 Borderline Personality Disorder

A pervasive pattern of instability of interpersonal relationships, self-image, and affects, and marked impulsivity beginning by early adulthood and present in a variety of contexts, as indicated by five (or more) of the following:

(1) frantic efforts to avoid real or imagined abandonment. *Note*: Do not include suicidal or self-mutilating behavior covered in Criterion 5.

(2) a pattern of unstable and intense interpersonal relationships characterized by alternating between extremes of idealization and devaluation

(3) identity disturbance: markedly and persistently unstable self-image or sense of self

(4) impulsivity in at least two areas that are potentially self-damaging (e.g., spending, sex, substance abuse, reckless driving, binge eating). *Note*: Do not include suicidal or self-mutilating behavior covered in Criterion 5.

(5) recurrent suicidal behavior, gestures, or threats, or self-mutilating behavior

(6) affective instability due to a marked reactivity of mood (e.g., intense episodic dysphoria, irritability, or anxiety usually lasting a few hours and only rarely more than a few days)

(7) chronic feelings of emptiness

(8) inappropriate, intense anger or difficulty controlling anger (e.g., frequent displays of temper, constant anger, recurrent physical fights)

(9) transient, stress-related paranoid ideation or severe dissociative symptoms

*Reprinted with permission from the *Diagnostic and Statistical Manual of Mental Disorders, Fourth Edition*. Copyright 1994 American Psychiatric Association.

derline pathology. At this phase, children lack object constancy and thus cannot integrate the good and bad aspects of themselves or their mothers. Neither can they separate from their mothers as they have yet to internalize a whole, soothing internalized usage of the mother to sustain them during her physical absence. Kernberg points to a disturbance in the mother's emotional availability during the rapprochement subphase that is attributable to the constitutional excess of aggression in the child, to maternal problems with parenting, or to both.

Masterson (1976) and Masterson and Klein (1990) implicate the rapprochement subphase, but emphasize the mother's behavior rather than the child's aggression. Typically a borderline herself, the mother is deeply conflicted about her children's growing up and becoming their own persons. Thus these children receive the message that if they grow up, something awful will happen to them or to their mothers, and that remaining dependent is the only way to maintain the maternal bond. This prospect of separation and individuation thus provokes "abandonment depression" in borderlines. No integration between a rewarding object unit and a withdrawing object unit is possible at this rapprochement subphase, accounting for the symptom of the borderline syndrome.

Adler's (1985) understanding of borderline pathology is influenced by Kohut (1971, 1977) and Fraiberg (1969), and is based on a deficit rather than a conflict model as with Kernberg. Inconsistency in maternal behavior and availability results in the borderline's failure to develop a "holding-nothing" internalized object. This accounts for feelings of emptiness, depressive tendencies, and oral rage. Furthermore, the borderline individual has difficulty with summoning up internal images of the natural nurturing figure in stressful situations. This cognitive deficit of evocative memory suggests a regression to a developmental age of between eight and 18 months. These inadequate resources leave the borderline prone to fragmentation of the self, which is accompanied by profound emptiness called "annihilation panic."

Biosocial Formulation

Millon (1981) views the borderline's lack of a clear, coherent sense of identity as central to the pathogenesis of this disorder. He believes that identity confusion or diffusion is the result of biopsychosocial factors that combine to impair a coherent sense of identity. Because of this central deficit, poorly coordinated actions, overmodulated affects, poorly controlled impulses, and a failure of consistent effort result. Thus the borderline individual depends on others for protection and reassurance, and is hypersensitive to the loss or separation of these supports. On the basis of this research, Millon (1981) and Millon and Everly (1985) contend that the borderline syndrome is essentially a more severe and regressed variant of the dependent, histrionic, or passive-aggressive personalty disorders. Biologically and temperamentally, borderline dependent individuals tend to exhibit a passive infantile pattern and to possess family histories marked by low energy levels. This pattern evokes parental warmth and overprotection, and they subsequently form strong attachments to and dependency on a single caregiver, which ultimately restricts their opportunity to learn the necessary skills for social independence and self-efficacy. This sets the stage for rejection by those on whom they have come to rely.

Borderline histrionic individuals more often have family histories characterized by high autonomic reactivity, and they exhibit hyper-responsiveness as a result of exposure to high levels of stimulation. Parental control tends to be exercised by contingent reinforcement patterns, and so these children feel competent and accepted only if their behavior is explicitly approved by others, and thus they "perform" to secure support, attention, and nurturance.

Borderline passive-aggressive individuals tend to have exhibited "difficult child" (Thomas & Chess, 1977) temperaments. As irritable, difficult-to-soothe infants, they likely received inconsistent responses from their caregivers—caring at times, harried and frustrated at other times, and even withdrawing. They might have been products of broken homes, and probably had a parent who modeled the erratic, vacillating, passive-aggressive behavior they display as adults.

Cognitive-Behavioral Formulations

According to Beck et al. (1990), three basic assumptions are noted in borderlines: "I am powerless and vulnerable," "I am inherently unacceptable," and "The world is dangerous and malevolent." Because of their inherent belief that they are helpless in a hostile world without a source of security, they vacillate between autonomy and dependence, without being able to rely on either. In addition, borderlines tend to display "dichotomous thinking," the tendency to evaluate experiences in mutually exclusive categories, all good or all bad, success or failure, trustworthy or deceitful. The combination of dichotomous thinking and basic assumptions is the basis of borderline emotion and behavior, including acting-out, self-destructive behaviors.

Young (1990) believes that "early maladaptive schemas" develop during childhood and result in maladaptive behavior patterns that reinforce these schemas. Schemas such as abandonment/loss ("I'll be alone forever. No one would live with me or want to be close to me if they really got to know me") and emotional deprivation ("No one is ever there to meet my needs, to be strong for me, to care for me") are believed to be common early maladaptive schemas in borderlines.

Linehan (1987) describes a behavioral formulation of borderline pathology. She claims that a dysfunction of emotional regulation is the core feature of borderline pathology, resulting in dramatic overreaction and impulsivity. This dysfunction is believed to be physiologically based and to be reinforced by significant others who discount their emotional experiences. Subsequently, borderline individuals develop little or no skill in emotion regulation. The combination of intense emotional responses, inadequate emotional regulation skills, impulsive behavior, and a disparaging self-attitude presages unrelenting crises with which they are unable to cope effectively, and overreliance on others. From a different behavioral perspective, Turkat (1990) believes that problem-solving deficits are the basis of borderline pathology.

Interpersonal Formulation

For Benjamin (1993), persons with borderline personality disorders typically grew up in a family marked by a chaotic, soap-opera lifestyle. Without these dilemmas, life was experienced as hollow, boring, and empty. Whether these chaotic dramas were blatant or were sequestered from public view, the borderline-to-be played a central role, resulting in the impulsivity, mood instability, and unpredictability characteristic of life without constancy. The developmental histories of these individuals often included traumatic abandonment experiences, the isolation of which was typically marked by physical or sexual abuse. This abuse-laden aloneness became inexorably linked with the notion that the borderline-to-be was a bad person. These abuse experiences "taught" the individual to shift from idealization to devaluation. And to the extent that the sexual abuse experiences were painful, they set the stage for self-mutilation, as pleasure became confused with pain during such episodes. Family norms dictated that autonomy was bad, whereas dependency on and sympathetic misery with the family were good. In movements toward independence, competence or happiness elicited self-sabotage. Furthermore, young borderline individuals learned from their families that misery, sickness, and debilitation draw forth love and concern from others. The adult consequence is that borderline-disordered individuals believe that caregivers and lovers secretly love misery. In short, there is a morbid fear of abandonment and a wish for protective nurturance, particularly from a lover or caregiver. Initially, friendly dependency on the nurturer gives way to hostile control when the person fails to deliver enough. Borderline individuals believe that significant others secretly like dependency and neediness, and a vicious introject attacks the self in the face of any signs of success or happiness.

Integrative Formulation

The following integrative formulation may be helpful in understanding how the borderline personality pattern is likely to have developed and to be maintained.

Biologically, borderlines can be understood in terms of the three main subtypes: borderline dependent, borderline histrionic, and borderline passive-aggressive. The temperamental style of the borderline dependent type is that of the passive infantile pattern (Millon, 1981). Millon hypothesized that low autonomic nervous system reactivity, plus an overprotective parenting style, facilitates restrictive interpersonal skills and a clinging relational style. The histrionic subtype is more likely to have had a hyperresponsive infantile pattern. Thus, because of high autonomic nervous system reactivity and increased parental stimulation and expectations for performance, the borderline histrionic pattern was likely to result. Finally, the temperamental style of the passive-aggressive borderline was likely to have been the "difficult child" type noted by Thomas and Chess (1977). This pattern, together with parental inconsistency, marks the affective irritability of the borderline passive-aggressive personality.

Psychologically, borderlines tend to view themselves, others, the world, and life's purpose in terms of the following themes. They view themselves by some variant of the theme: "I don't know who I am or where I'm going." In short, their identity problems involve gender, career, loyalties, and values, while their self-esteem fluctuates with each thought or feeling about their self-identity. Borderlines tend to view their world with some variant of the theme: "People are great; no, they are not"; "Having goals is good; no, it's not"; or "If life doesn't go my way, I can't tolerate it." As such, they are likely to conclude: "Therefore, keep all options open. Don't commit to anything. Reverse roles and vacillate in your thinking and feeling when under attack." The defensive operations utilized by the person with a borderline personality disorder are denial, splitting, primitive idealization, projective identification, omnipotence, and devaluation (Shulman, 1982).

Socially, predictable patterns of parenting and environmental factors can be noted for the borderline personality disorder. The parenting style differs depending on the subtype. For example, in the dependent subtype, overprotectiveness characterizes parenting, whereas in the histrionic subtype, a demanding parenting style is more evident, and an inconsistent parenting style is noted in the passive-aggressive subtype. But because the borderline personality is a syndromal elaboration and deterioration of the less severe dependent, histrionic, or passive-aggressive personality disorders, the family of origin in the borderline subtypes of these disorders is likely to be much more dysfunctional, increasing the likelihood the child will have learned various self-defeating coping strategies. The parental injunction is likely to have been, "If you grow up and leave me, bad things will happen to me (parent)."

This borderline pattern is confirmed, reinforced, and perpetuated by the following individual and systems factors: diffuse identity, impulsive vacillation, and self-defeating coping strategies leading to aggressive acting out, which leads to more chaos, which leads to the experience of depersonalization, increased dysphoria, or self-mutilation to achieve some relief. This leads to further reconfirmation of beliefs about the self and the world, as well as reinforcement of the behavioral and interpersonal patterns (Sperry & Mosak, 1993).

Table 4.3
Characteristics of Borderline Personality Disorder

1. Behavioral appearance	"Hemophiliacs" of emotion; resentful, impulsive, acting out; helpless, dysphoric, empty "void"; irregular circadian rhythms (sleep–wake, etc.)
2. Interpersonal behavior	Paradoxical—idealizing and clinging vs. devaluing and oppositional; rejection sensitivity, abandonment depression; separation anxiety as prime motivator; role reversal
3. Cognitive style	Inflexible, rigid abstracting, grandiosity and idealization, splitting; reasons by analogy—doesn't learn from experience; external loss of control—blaming; poorly developed evocative memory
4. Feeling style	Extreme lability of mood and affect
5. Parental injunction/environment	"If you grow up, bad things will happen to me (parent)." Overprotective or demanding or inconsistent parenting
6. Biological/temperament	*Dependent type*: passive infantile pattern→low autonomic nervous system reactivity (+) parental overprotectiveness→ restrictive interpersonal skills and pleasing, clinging style; *histrionic type*: hyperresponsive infantile pattern—high automatic reactivity (+) high parental stimulation, and demand for child to "perform." *Passive-aggressive type*: "difficult" infantile pattern→affect irritability (+) parental inconsistency
7. Self view	"I don't know who I am or where I'm going." Identity problems involving gender, career, loyalties, and values. Self-esteem fluctuates with current emotion.
8. World view	"People are great, no they're not. Having goals is good; no, it's not. If life doesn't go my way, I can't tolerate it. Therefore, keep all options open. Don't commit to anything. Reverse roles when under attack."
9. Self and system perpetuant	Self-defeating coping strategies—particularly "reversal" (i.e., from submissiveness to aggressiveness)→ more chaos→ depersonalization, brief psychotic episodes, increased dysphoria or self-mutilation to achieve relief→ reconfirmation of core beliefs→ reinforcement of borderline style

ASSESSMENT OF BORDERLINE PERSONALITY DISORDER

Several sources of information are useful in establishing a diagnosis and treatment plan for personality disorders. Observation, collateral information, and psychological testing are important adjuncts to the patient's self-report in the clinical interview. This section briefly describes some characteristic observations that the clinician makes and the nature of the rapport likely to develop in initial encounters with specific personality-disordered individuals. Characteristic response patterns on various objective (i.e., MMPI-2 and MCMI-II) and projective (i.e., Rorschach and TAT) tests are also described.

Interviewing patients with borderline personality disorders presents a special challenge because of their instability and ambivalence. Instability or lability is noted in their moods, goals, and rapport with the clinician. Instability regarding rapport is handled by empathically focusing on it. This is done by directing the discussion, keeping the discussion on track, and curbing diversions and outbursts. Asking open-ended questions is preferable to seeking precise answers to closed-ended pointed questions. Instability is also processed by separating it as a pathological part that needs to be explored. Since it also affects rapport, the clinician must continually acknowledge its presence and effect. The result is that these patients become less defensive and more willing to disclose, thus furthering rapport.

Dealing with ambivalence requires confronting their contradictions, while at the same time exhibiting an understanding of their ambivalent feelings. Therapeutic confrontation illustrates their splitting and projective identification and moderates overidealization or devaluation. It further helps these individuals to realize that their ambivalence results from a perceived lack of support and understanding of their mothers, which they allow to profoundly influence their sense of well-being (Othmer & Othmer, 1989).

The Minnesota Multiphasic Personality Inventory (MMPI-2), the Millon Clinical Multiaxial Inventory (MCMI-II), the Rorschach Psychodiagnostic Test, and the Thematic Apperception Test (TAT) can be useful in diagnosing the borderline personality disorder, as well as the borderline personality style or trait.

On the MMPI-2, elevations on scales 2 (Depression), 4 (Psychothemia), and 8 (Schizophrenia) are common. Scales O (Social Introversion) and K (Correction) tend to be high; F (Frequency) is typically low. If emotional dysregulation—particularly of anger—is prominent, scale 6 (Paranoia) will be high. Although relatively rare, a 2–6 (Depression–Paranoia) 6–2 profile is associated with borderline pathology (Meyer, 1993).

On the MCMI-II, elevation on scale C (Borderline) is most likely, and a concurrent elevation on scale 8A (Passive-aggressive) is also likely. Elevations on such clinical scales as A (Anxiety), H (Somatoform), N (Bipolar—Manic) and/or D (Dysthymia) can be expected (Choca, Shanely, & Denburg, 1992).

On the Rorschach, illogical and fabulized combinations (i.e., "a horse's head with two sea horses growing out of his ears" for card 10) are common (Swiercinsky, 1985). Such responses are most likely on cards 10.9 and 2.

On the TAT, "primitive splitting" may be noted in characters that are judged as all bad (i.e., devils), in characters wherein only one side of the personality is admitted to or portrayed, or when good–bad characteristics are juxtaposed incongruously. Separation anxiety themes, extreme portrayals of affect, and acting out rather than delayed gratification are not uncommon (Bellak, 1993).

TREATMENT APPROACHES AND INTERVENTIONS

Treatment Considerations

Included in the differential diagnosis of the borderline personality disorder are these other Axis II personality disorders: passive-aggressive personality disorder, histrionic personality disorder, dependent personality disorder, and the schizotypal personality disorder. The most common Axis I syndromes associated with the personality disorder are generalized anxiety disorder, panic disorder, and dysthymia. In addition, other syndromes may be brief reactive psychoses, schizoaffective disorder, hypochondriasis, or the dissociative disorders, especially psychogenic fugue.

The borderline personality disorder may be the most common Axis II presentation seen in both the public sector and private practice. And it can be among the most difficult and frustrating conditions to treat. Clinical experience suggests that it is important to assess the individual for overall level of functioning and treatment readiness in making decisions about treatment approaches, modalities, and strategies.

INDIVIDUAL PSYCHOTHERAPIES

Many consider individual psychotherapy to be the cornerstone of treatment for the borderline personality disorder. Although there are widely divergent opinions on the appropriateness or efficacy of the various individual psychotherapeutic approaches, there is consensus on some general principles. Waldinger (1986) describes five points of consensus on treating the borderline personality. First, the therapist must be active in identifying, confronting, and directing the patient's behaviors during sessions. Second, a stable treatment environment must be afforded in terms of setting and maintaining limits and boundaries, scheduling, payment of fees, and role expectations of patient and clinician. Third, connection between the patient's actions and feelings in the present need to be established. Fourth, self-destructive behavior must be made ungratifying. And fifth, careful attention must be paid to countertransference feelings.

Regardless of the specific psychotherapeutic approach utilized, the literature indicates that treatment of the borderline patient is difficult, countertransference problems are common, and the results are uneven (Gunderson, 1989). Some borderline patients have negative therapeutic reactions, and others experience untoward effects of individual psychotherapy. In some instances, these patients should not be afforded individual treatment. Frances, Clarkin, and Perry (1984) offer the "no treatment option," along with specific criteria for its use. Nevertheless, when treatment is indicated, attention to the patient's needs and expectations for treatment and efforts to match and tailor treatment are essential in maximizing treatment outcomes.

This section describes various psychodynamic, cognitive-behavioral, and interpersonal approaches.

Psychodynamic Psychotherapy

Here is a brief outline of various psychodynamic approaches to the borderline personality: psychoanalytic psychotherapy, supportive psychotherapy, and short-term dynamic psychotherapy.

Psychoanalytic Psychotherapy
There are basically two psychoanalytic opinions regarding the treatment of the borderline patients based on the role of early interpretation and the management of negative transference. One view is that confrontation must occur early in the course of treatment and that interpretation of primitive transference must be made in here-and-now situations. The other view is that early interpretations of the aggressive theme are ineffective, and possibly disruptive. Kernberg (1984) and Masterson (1976), among others, espouse the first view, whereas Chessick (1982), Buie and Adler (1982), and others advocate the second. Nevertheless, both views agree that personality reconstruction is the goal of treatment, requiring three or more sessions a week for a minimum of four years.

Masterson (1976) and Masterson and Klein (1989) have elegantly described the psychotherapeutic process with borderline patients.

Supportive psychotherapy is differentiated from reconstructive psychotherapy. The goal of reconstructive psychotherapy is to work through the abandonment depression—feelings of depression, anger and rage, fear, guilt, passivity and helplessness, emptiness and void that follow a recent experience of separation and loss—associated with the original separation–individuation phase. This leads to the achievement of ego autonomy and the transformation of split-object relations into whole-object relations and at the split ego into a whole ego. Three stages of psychotherapy are noted by Masterson: the testing phase, in which the clinician utilizes confrontation or communicative matching to support the patient's emerging individuation as the principal technique; the working-through phase; and the separation phase.

The expected outcome of such treatment is not only reduction in impulsive behavior and other regressive reactions to stressors, but also improved stability in interpersonal relationships. Such personality reconstruction allows the individual to function normally or on a neurotic level (Gunderson, 1989).

Supportive Psychotherapy
From a dynamic perspective, supportive psychotherapy is less intensive and regressive than is psychoanalytic psychotherapy or psychoanalysis. The goals of supportive therapy with borderline individuals are principally to improve their adaptation to daily life and to reduce their self-destructive responses to interpersonal stressors (Kernberg, 1984).

The basic techniques of supportive psychotherapy consist of exploring the patients' primitive defenses in the here-and-now for the purpose of helping them achieve control by nonanalytic means, and fostering a better adaptation to reality by helping them become more aware of the disorganizing effect of their defensive operations. Manifest and suppressed transferences—rather than unconscious and repressed transferences—are explored and utilized in order to classify the related interpersonal problems the patient faces (Kernberg, 1984).

Such supportive psychotherapy commonly is utilized with moderately and lower functioning borderline outpatients. Typically, sessions are scheduled weekly and may continue for several years. The results of the Menninger outcome study suggest that supportive treatment is able to bring about the basic personality changes that were expected only from reconstructive dynamic psychotherapy (Wallerstein, 1986). So, despite Kernberg's (1984) characterization of supportive psychotherapy as "a treatment of last resort," it can be a potent intervention.

Klein (1989a) describes two types of supportive treatment for lower functioning borderlines. In the first, confrontative psychotherapy, the treatment process involves confronting resistances that maintain maladaptive behaviors until they become ego dystonic. A therapeutic alliance takes the place of transference acting out. Treatment also involves the implementation of adaptive modes of dealing with underlying affects, such as new patterns replacing previous self-destructive behaviors and defenses. Unlike reconstructive psychotherapy, this approach does not facilitate the patient's working through abandonment depression. Its goals are limited to increasing the patient's capacity to work to achieve some consistency in interpersonal relationships.

Klein (1989a) also describes an approach to "counseling" with very low functioning borderline patients. This approach is the treatment of choice for patients with a history of repeated early abuse; neglect or separation trauma; repeated, severe psychiatric regressive episodes; or repeated life-threatening suicidal or homicidal actions. The goal of this treatment is to reduce anger, anxiety, and the depressive affects that persistently interfere with the patient's capacity to function adaptively. The counselor serves as an auxiliary ego for the patient, and utilizes a combination of such techniques as reality testing, encouragement, direction, problem solving, and medication.

Short-Term Psychotherapy

Although it was previous assumed that borderline patients were unfit for short-term dynamic psychotherapy, it now appears that short-term and time-limited approaches have some utility with selected patients. In as few as 10 to 20 sessions, treatment can be focused on specific relational or situational problems. And because the focus is so specific, the likelihood of having a regressive transference develop is limited. This approach may be suitable for borderline patients who present with concerns about being engulfed, overwhelmed, or too dependent. It may also be useful for those who have a history of terminating more regressive treatment. Furthermore, it may serve as a springboard for moving into long-term therapy.

Klein (1989b) describes a short-term treatment protocol for borderline patients. The goals are containment (i.e., they come to recognize, control, and contain their propensity to act out); learning (i.e., that emerging affects that covered their defenses can and must be verbalized rather than acted out); and adaptation (i.e., they channel their energies associated with these affects into adaptive and sublimated behavior and expressions). This short-term approach follows Masterson's model, except that the frequency of sessions is limited and confrontation is the principal technique utilized, although clarification, interpretation, and communicative matching are sometimes needed. Sessions are scheduled only once or twice a week for a year or less, and day-to-day problems of adaptation and healthy defenses are the focus of treatment.

Cognitive-Behavioral Approach

According to Beck et al. (1990), the cognitive therapy approach has significant advantages over other approaches in the treatment of patients with borderline personality disorders. Basically, completion of cognitive therapy is possible in 1 1/2 to 2 1/2 years, as compared with psychoanalytically oriented therapies, which typically require five to seven years (Masterson, 1981).

Establishing a collaborative working relationship is the very challenging first step in the treatment process. Since trust and intimacy are major issues for these individuals, taking a collaborative, strategic approach based on guided discovery is suggested. Explicitly acknowledging and accepting the individual's difficulty in trusting the therapist; communicating clearly, assertively, and honestly; following through on agreements; and behaving in a consistently trustworthy manner provide the individual with evidence on which trust can be based. Furthermore, setting limits, including specifying a treatment contract, is advised. An initial focus on concrete behavioral goals is useful in reducing the impact of the borderline individual's difficulty with intimacy and trust. Many of these individuals find it less threatening to work on issues for which little introspection is required, and where the focus is on behavior rather than on feelings or thoughts. Not surprisingly, a major focus in cognitive therapy is changing maladaptive schemas. Borderline individuals believe that the world is a dangerous place, that they are helpless, and that they are inherently flawed in a way that inevitably leads to rejection and abandonment by others. It is suggested that these beliefs must be gradually challenged by "chipping away" at them, by testing expectancies against previous experience, by developing behavioral experiences to test expectancies, and by developing new competencies and coping skills. These individuals must learn to challenge dichotomous thinking, both during and between sessions, as decreased dichotomous thinking often results in decreased mood lability and impulsivity. Behavioral interventions, such as self-instructional training (Meichenbaum, 1977), may be useful in further reducing self-destructive impulsive behaviors.

Noncompliance with treatment is not an uncommon problem with borderline individuals, and often the reason is fear of change. Since they assume the world is dangerous and they have a low tolerance for ambiguity, they find change, including growth in the course of treatment, threatening. Addressing change openly, examining risks and benefits, planning changes as a series of small steps, and not pressing for change too quickly are recommended. Fears about termination of treatment evoke abandonment and rejection schemas, which must be carefully addressed. In summary, the cognitive therapy of patients with borderline personality disorders begins by developing a collaborative working relationship of trust, and then focuses on modulating moods, impulses, and behavior with cognitive-behavioral methods, setting the stage so that such basic schemas as abandonment, defectiveness, incompetence, and mistrust can be modified and changed.

In line with Turkat's (1990) formulation that the basic issue for borderlines is problem-solving deficiencies, he proposes a treatment methodology involving several strategies—basic problem-solving training, concept-formation training, categorization management, and processing-speed management.

Interpersonal Approach

For Benjamin (1993), psychotherapeutic interventions with persons with borderline personality disorders can be planned and evaluated in terms of whether they enhance collaboration, facilitate learning about maladaptive patterns and their roots, block these patterns, enhance the will to change, and effectively encourage new patterns.

Benjamin offers a number of observations on facilitating collaboration. She insists that therapists offer these individuals a contract for strength building rather than in enabling regression. A collaboration based on strength building must emphasize, in sessions as well as in telephone calls or in the clinic lobby, that the mutual goal is to build on strengths so that these individuals can pull themselves back together. The collaboration must be against "it," their destructive pattern. Healthy collaboration further requires that transference and countertransference disasters be avoided by setting firm physical and verbal boundaries. Benjamin cautions that the treatment approach she advocates is not appropriate for those who are unable to agree to a contract in strength building.

Borderline individuals need to learn to recognize that perceived abandonment sets off a chain of self-destructive patterns. Thy are likely to relinquish self-mutilation, self-sabotage, and homicidal or suicidal acting out if they can "divorce" their internalized abusive attachment figures. Essentially, they must give up the desire to be affirmed by these internalized representations. This occurs by developing a dislike of those figures, or by developing a superseding attachment to someone more constructive, such as the clinician. Once these tasks are achieved, the focus of treatment shifts to facilitating new learning. The basic goal is learning how to give and take autonomy while remaining friendly. Benjamin recommends standard treatments for facilitating personal growth.

GROUP THERAPY

Data on the efficacy of group therapy for the treatment of personality disorders are rather "soft." There are many case reports, and even a few controlled studies, but no randomized clinical trials, except for the borderline personality disorder—for which there are numerous reports of cases and clinical trials, and even of one randomized clinical trial. Moreover, there is a general consensus that group therapy, under specified conditions, has enormously therapeutic efficacy. This section reviews both dynamic and behavioral group approaches, and highlights some representative research studies.

The psychodynamic group literature on borderline personality begins in the 1950s. There is general consensus that group dynamic therapy can be a useful adjunct to individual dynamic therapy, but that it cannot be the only treatment (Hulse, 1958; Slavson, 1964; Day & Semrad, 1971; Horowitz, 1980). Horowitz (1980) cautions that borderline patients require individual psychotherapy to support them throughout group-engendered stress and to integrate the affects the group provokes in them. Furthermore, without individual psychotherapy, premature termination from group therapy is likely. However, Pines (1975) contends that concurrent dynamic individual psychotherapy is not necessary because the group process itself is a potent holding environment capable of containing primitive impulses and projections. Horowitz (1977) maintains that the individual psychotherapist should not function as group therapist so as to reduce the possibility of jealousy and fantasies of favoritism among other group members.

Most writers on dynamic group therapy for borderlines prefer heterogeneous to homogeneous groups. They insist that borderline patients are more effectively treated in groups consisting of higher functioning individuals with neuroses and other personality disorders (Day & Semrad, 1971; Horowitz, 1977; Stone & Weissman, 1984). There is, however, outcome research that supports the use of homogeneous groups in which all patients have diagnoses of borderline personality disorders (O'Leary, Turner, Gardner, et al., 1991; Finn & Shakir, 1990; Linehan, Armstrong, Suarez, et al., 1991).

The advantages of dynamic group therapy include "dilution of intense transference" (Horowitz, 1980), which results from the presence of multiple transferential objects, instead of the single all-encompassing individual clinician. Rage instead is diluted and directed toward other group members. Borderline patients also find it easier to accept feedback and confrontation from group peers than from a therapist. Groups also provide many opportunities to understand and master such borderline defenses as splitting and projective identification.

There are some disadvantages and difficulties with group treatment of borderline patients. First, these patients may be easily scapegoated because of their primitive manner of expression. Second, they may feel deprived amid the competition of other group members for the group leader's nurturance. And they may maintain a certain distance in the group because of their privacy attachment to their individual psychotherapist (Gabbard, 1994).

Dynamically oriented groups with borderlines tend to span the continuum from ego psychology (O'Leary et al., 1991; Finn & Shakir, 1990) to self psychology (Harwood, 1992).

Behavioral group therapies for borderline patients focus less on underlying explanations for the symptomatic behavior and more on helping the patients acquire the specific skills necessary to control their affects, reduce their cognitive distortions and projective identifications, and find alternatives to self-destructive behaviors. Linehan (1983, 1987, 1993) provides a manual-guided strategy for the treatment of self-destructive behavior and impulsivity called "dialectical behavior therapy." Geared primarily to chronically parasuicidal borderline women patients, the treatment strategies and interventions have applicability to more highly functioning individuals. The group session employs didactic skill training and behavioral rehearsal techniques directed at dependency and other interpersonal patterns, as well as at improving affect tolerance. These twice-weekly sessions for one year are complemented with weekly individual counseling.

There has been some noteworthy research with borderlines in group treatment that will be briefly highlighted. Nehls (1991) and Nehls and Diamond (1993) report process and outcome data on group therapy of borderline patients in a homogeneous treatment format. The group was highly structured, although group members defined their own treatment goals. Patient outcomes included decreased depression and hostility, which was associated largely with two interventions: providing and seeking information. Dick and Wooff (1986) reported data on a time-limited dynamic group therapy with heterogeneous groups containing a number of borderline patients. The group met daily for 12 weeks. A one-year follow-up showed an 82 percent reduction in the use of psychiatric services as compared with a control group of untreated patients, and a three-year follow-up showed that the gains had been maintained. Finally, Linehan et al. (1991) report the only randomized clinical trial to date. Parasuicidal female borderline patients were randomly assigned to dialectical behavior therapy groups or traditional community treatment for a one-year-period. Those in behavioral groups had fewer incidents of parasuicide, were more likely to remain in individual therapy, and had fewer inpatient psychiatric days than did those in traditional treatment. A manual-guided approach called relationship management psychotherapy is a time-limited group approach that is being compared with open-ended individual dynamic psychotherapy in a randomized clinical trial. The study is still in progress, but preliminary results are encouraging (Clarkin, Marzaliali, & Munroe-Blum, 1991).

MARITAL/FAMILY THERAPY

Families of borderline patients often exhibit severe pathology, which may be of etiological significance. Borderline patients' parents have a high incidence of affective disorders, alcoholism, antisocial personality disorder, and borderline personality disorder or traits. The parental relationship is usually characterized by neglect and overprotectiveness. Family therapy can be useful, and in some instances is necessary, in maintaining borderline patients in outpatient psychotherapy. This is particularly the case when borderline patients remain financially or emotional dependent on their parents.

Family therapy with borderlines has been developed along at least three theoretical lines. The first is the psychodynamic, particularly in terms of object relations and systems theory. Everett, Halperin, Volgy, and Wissler (1989) present the most complete discussion of this approach in their book, *Treating the Borderline Family: A Systemic Approach.* They specify five treatment goals: increasing the family's ability to reduce the systemic splitting process; increasing family members' capacities for owning split-off objects and moving toward interacting with others as a "whole person"; reducing oppositional and stereotypic behavior of all family members; "resetting" external boundaries for both unclear and intergenerational systems; "resetting" internal boundaries for spousal, parent–child, and sibling subtypes, permitting a clearer alliance between the parents and limiting reciprocal intrusiveness of children and parents. Five treatment strategies for accomplishing these goals in an outpatient family treatment setting are development and maintenance of a therapeutic structure, reality testing in the family, interactional disengagement, intervention in the intergenerational system, and solidification of the marital alliance and sibling subsystem.

Another treatment orientation is the structural family approach developed by Minuchin (1974). Schane and Kovel (1988) describe severe borderline pathology in terms of a spouse subsystem that is internally overinvolved and contemporarily distant and disengaged from the old subsystem. In effect, borderline women have a systems equivalent of object splitting, wherein family subsystems are organized around dichotomous extremes:

collusion and sabotage, loyalty and scapegoating, inclusion and rejection, nurturance and neglect, and symbiosis and abandonment. It is this structural pattern of family interaction that is the focus of systemic change. Lachar (1992) provides an extensive discussion of an integrated object-relations and self-psychology approach to the marital treatment of the borderline patient. She presents a detailed treatment protocol and several case reports that illustrate this method.

A third option is the relationship enhancement therapy approach for borderline families and couples. Relationship enhancement, developed by Guerney (1977), integrates social skills training, psychodynamic principles, and interpersonal therapy techniques. Since borderline patients have major deficits in self-differentiation and communication, the relationship enhancement's focus on skill building in some areas seems promising within couple and family settings, particularly for mild to moderately dysfunctional borderline patients (Waldo & Harman, 1993). The clinician functions largely as a coach to develop the necessary relational skills, usually in two-hour sessions. Waldo and Harman report a case of time-limited intervention that was successful. A 12-month follow-up showed that the changes had been maintained.

MEDICATION

A full gamut of psychotropic medications have been employed in the treatment of borderline patients, including low-dose antipsychotics, tricyclic antidepressants, anticonvulsants, and, most recently, selective serotonin reuptake inhibitors. Given that the diagnosis of borderline personality disorder encompasses a heterogeneous group of patients, often with intractable symptoms, both clinicians and patients have held high—and even magical—expectations for medication as a cure or, at the very least, as a palliative. Not surprisingly, the pharmacological treatment of borderline pathology can be difficult and frustrating for both clinician and patient.

The basic treatment strategy has been to match a medication to specific target symptoms. Recent pharmacological and neurobiological research suggests that the borderline disorder encompasses three clusters of symptoms: affective instability, impulsive aggressivity, and transient psychotic phenomena (Cocarro & Kavoussi, 1991). It appears that affective instability is related to brain abnormalities in adrenergic and cholinergic systems. It has been shown that such agents as lithium carbonate and carbamazepine are effective in modulating affects. Abnormalities in central nervous system serotonergic function resulting in impulsivity seem to respond to serotonergic agents such as fluoxetine (Prozac). Finally, abnormalities in central dopaminergic systems may account for transient psychotic symptoms.

Thus low-dose antipsychotics have been shown to be effective with this symptom cluster.

The possible efficacy of serotonin reuptake inhibitors specifically with borderline pathology, such as dysphoria and impulsive-aggressive behavior, has been the subject of a number of clinical trials. Fluoxetine (Prozac) appears to be effective in treating symptoms related to depressed mood and impulsive aggressivity (Cocarro, 1993). Markowitz, Colabrese, Schulz, and Meltzer (1991) report similar results in a prospective, nonblinded study. Double-blind, placebo-controlled trials should help confirm the efficacy of this class of medication for borderline pathology. However, there are some potential complications or disadvantages with pharmacotherapy in the treatment of borderline patients. First is the matter of noncompliance, related either to side effects or to secondary gain. Medications can serve as a leverage to control the prescribing clinician or other caregivers. Demands for frequent changes in the dose or type of medication, overdosing, and failure to take the medication as it was prescribed are ways of transference acting out. Second, although borderline patients may appear to others to have improved while on medication, they may report that they feel worse, or vice versa. Gunderson (1989) suggests that this apparent paradox may come about if the patient believes that symptomatic improvement will result in undesirable consequences, such as loss or abandonment of dependent gratifications.

Perhaps the most clinically useful contribution to the literature is that by Klein (1989c) who skillfully describes the integration of pharmacotherapy into an individual psychotherapy context. He provides three guidelines for the effective utilization of medication: careful attention to diagnostic precision, evaluation of objective signs rather than subjective symptoms when determining when and which medication to use, and controlled awareness of the risks of therapeutic medication. Seven case histories illustrate these guidelines. Klein's chapter should be required reading for both medical and nonmedical clinicians involved in the treatment of borderline patients.

COMBINED AND INTEGRATED TREATMENT APPROACHES

There is considerable consensus that combined treatment is essential, or at least preferable, for borderline pathology, given its severity and apparent treatment resistance. Clearly, differences exist between the prognosis and treatability of the highly functioning borderline (i.e., GAF over 65) and the low functioning borderline (i.e., GAF below 45). Treatment success using only traditional individual psychoanalytic psychotherapy may be possible with the highest functioning borderline individual, but is not likely with the lower functioning patients. In line with the basic premise of this book, the lower the patient's functioning, motivation, and readiness for treatment, the more that treatment must be integrated and combined.

The most common recommendations for combined treatment is to prescribe both individual therapy and group therapy. There is currently no consensus on which theoretical approaches to combine or whether they should be combined or sequenced. The earliest recommendations for combined treatment was by Tacbacnik (1965), who advocated concurrent dynamic individual psychotherapy and dynamic group therapy. Horowitz (1977, 1980), however, advocates sequencing dynamic group and individual therapy, in which the group experience prepares the patient to utilize individual therapy productively. Clarkin et al. (1991) also recommend combined individual and group modalities, but favor individual behavior treatment with long-term manual-guided group treatment.

Others recommend combining individual therapy and family therapy, including Kernberg (1984), who describes the indications for concurrent as well as sequential utilization of these modalities.

Berger (1987) recommends combined psychotherapy and pharmacotherapy because these individuals are difficult to treat with only one modality. He notes that combined treatment can be complicated by the borderline's tendency to idealize one treatment and negate the other. Koenigsberg (1993) offers a very thoughtful review of combining medications and psychotherapy, highlighting the indications for and contraindications to this treatment decision. He also describes the complications inherent in a combined treatment strategy, but adds that these can be addressed by special structuring of treatment, attention to countertransference issues, and vigilance for splitting. Koenigsberg contends that combining medication and psychotherapy has considerable value for seriously symptomatic patients, those prone to treatment noncompliance, or those who are likely to undergo intractable affective storms and psychotic regression.

Lazarus (1985), the developer of multimodal therapy, endorses the combined use of several modalities, concurrently or sequentially, for a variety of difficult patients, including borderline individuals. Vaccani (1989) describes treating the alcohol-abusing borderline personality with psychotherapy, family therapy, group therapy, and attendance at Alcoholics Anonymous meetings. Nehls and Diamond (1993) describe the modalities for lower functioning borderlines in a community-based setting. These modalities, which are coordinated and continuous, include individual therapy, group therapy, medication, drug and alcohol services, psychosocial rehabilitation, crisis intervention, and use of crisis houses.

CHAPTER 5

Dependent Personality Disorder

The concept of dependency is well established in the psychological literature. Whereas early psychoanalytic theory emphasized the "oral character" and structural basis of dependency, social learning theory considered
dependency to be acquired by learning and experience, and ethological
theory posited that attachment or affectional bonding is the basis for dependency. All three theories have contributed to the concept of dependent
personality disorder as defined by DSM. The basic feature of the disorder
is abnormal dependency causing subjective distress and/or functional impairment. However, the definition and criteria have changed in the different versions of DSM. In DSM-I, passive dependency personality was
characterized by helplessness, denial, and indecisiveness, and was considered a subtype of the passive-aggressive personality. DSM-II listed passive
dependent personality as "Other Personality Disorders of Specific Types"
and gave no description or criteria. Convinced that a "passive-dependent"
type was needed to counterbalance the "active-dependent" or histrionic
personality disorder, dependent personality disorder was added to DSM-
III (Hirschfield, Shea, & Weise, 1991), which gave three criteria (expanded
to nine in DSM-III-R), of which the essential feature was a pervasive pattern of dependent and submissive behavior. DSM-IV emphasizes the excessive need to be taken care of, leading to submissive and clinging behavior
and fear of separation.

No reliable data are currently available on the prevalence of this disorder. A Canadian study in 1963 suggested that 2.5 percent of the population could meet the criteria (Stone, 1993), but this rate seems very low. The disorder is more common among women than among men (Gunderson, 1989). In women the dependent style often takes the form of submissiveness, whereas in men, it is more likely to be autocratic, as when the husband and boss depends on his wife and secretary to perform essential tasks he himself cannot accomplish. In either case, this disorder is likely to lead to anxiety and depression when the dependent relationship is threatened.

This chapter describes the characteristic features of the dependent personality disorder and its related personality style. Five clinical formulations of the disorder and psychological assessment indicators are highlighted. A variety of treatment approaches, modalities, and intervention strategies are also described.

CHARACTERISTICS OF THE DEPENDENT
PERSONALITY STYLE AND DISORDER

The dependent personality can be thought of as spanning a continuum from healthy to pathological, with the dependent personality style at the healthy end and the dependent personality disorder at the pathological end. Table 5.1 compares and contrasts differences between the dependent style and the disorder.

Dependent personality disorder can be recognized by the following behavioral and interpersonal, cognitive, and affective styles.

The behavioral and interpersonal styles of dependent personalities are characterized by docility, passivity, and nonassertiveness. In interpersonal relations, they tend to be pleasing, self-sacrificing, and clinging, and constantly require the assurance of others. Their compliance and reliance on others lead to a subtle demand that others assume responsibility for major areas of their lives.

The cognitive style of dependent personalities is characterized by suggestibility. They easily adopt a Pollyannaish attitude toward life. Furthermore, they tend to minimize difficulties, and because of their naiveté, are readily persuadable and others easily take advantage of them. In short, this style of thinking is uncritical and unperceptive.

Their emotional or affective style is characterized by insecurity and anxiousness. Because they lack self-confidence, they experience considerable discomfort at being alone. They tend to be preoccupied with the fear of abandonment and of the disapproval of others. Their mood tends to be one of anxiety or fearfulness, as well as having a somber or sad quality.

Table 5.1
Comparison of the Dependent Personality Style and Disorder

Personality Style	*Personality Disorder*
• Seek out the opinions and advice of others when making decisions, but ultimately make their own decisions.	• Unable to make everyday decisions, seeking an excessive amount of advice or reassurance from others; allow others to make most of their important decisions.
• Carefully promote harmony with important persons in their life by being polite, agreeable, and tactful.	• Agree with people when they believe they are wrong, because of fear of being rejected.
• Although they respect authority and prefer the role of team member, they can initiate and complete tasks on their own.	• Have difficulty initiating projects or doing things on their own.
• Thoughtful of and good at pleasing others; occasionally, they will endure personal discomfort in accomplishing a good deed for the key people in their lives.	• Volunteer to do things that are unpleasant or demeaning in order to get other people to like them.
• Tend to prefer the company of one or more persons to being alone.	• Feel uncomfortable or helpless when alone or go to great lengths to avoid being alone.
• Tend to be strongly committed to relationships and work hard to sustain them.	• Feel devastated or helpless when close relationships end, and frequently are preoccupied with fears of being abandoned.
• Can take corrective action in response to criticism.	• Easily hurt by criticism or disapproval.

The following two case examples further illustrate the difference between the dependent personality disorder (Ms. C.) and the dependent personality style (Mr. B.).

Case Study: Dependent Personality Disorder

Ms. C. is a 38-year-old, single woman with panic symptoms that had begun approximately three years earlier. Once the panic attacks began, Ms. C. moved back into her parents' home and has become nearly totally housebound, fearing that "panic could strike any time." She described both of her parents as caring, concerned, and "my best friends," on whom she is overly reliant. She looks to them to support her financially and emotionally, and to make decisions for her. Ms. C. has also become progressively habituated to the Valium that she was prescribed for panic symptoms.

Case Study: Dependent Personality Style

Mr. B. has been a social worker at a foster-care agency for the past seven years. He finds his job fulfilling and is well liked by the other staff members, as well as the children and prospective parents with whom he works. He is a very concerned, caring, and gentle person. A year earlier, he had begun dating Sandra L., one of the pediatricians who consults to the agency. Their relationship has been happy and fulfilling for both of them, probably because of Mr. B.'s efforts. He can not get over the fact that a doctor would be interested in being with him, and he expresses his appreciation in numerous ways. He can not spend enough time with her, or do enough things for her. He idealizes her, makes every effort to make her feel comfortable and secure, and regularly seeks her opinions and advice. Yet he insists that he has a mind of his own; after much deliberation and soul searching, he bought an expensive sports car even though Sandra thought it was extravagant.

DSM-IV Description and Criteria

Table 5.2 presents the DSM-IV description and criteria.

FORMULATIONS OF DEPENDENT PERSONALITY DISORDER

Psychodynamic Formulation

Early psychoanalytic writers posited that dependent personalities were formed in the oral phase of psychosexual development. Contemporary formulations view the development of dependency as a function of parental—particularly maternal—overinvolvement and intrusiveness throughout all phases of development. These individuals often present histories of parental reward for maintaining loyalty, and subtle parental rejection whenever they attempted separation and independence. They would react with crying and clinging behavior, while being immobilized by fear and dread of abandonment. Their submissive stance is the result of multiply determined unconscious factors. Gabbard (1990) notes that dependent personalities typically seek to be cared for by others because of their underlying anxiety, which often masks aggression. Dependency thus

Table 5.2
DSM-IV Description and Criteria for Dependent Personality Disorder*

301.6 Dependent Personality Disorder

A pervasive and excessive need to be taken care of, that leads to submissive and clinging behavior and fears of separation, beginning by early adulthood and present in a variety of contexts, as indicated by five (or more) of the following:

(1) has difficulty in making everyday decisions without an excessive amount of advice and reassurance from others

(2) needs others to assume responsibility for most major areas of his or her life

(3) has difficulty expressing disagreement with others because of fear of loss of support or approval. *Note*: Do not include realistic fears of retribution.

(4) has difficulty initiating projects or doing things on his or her own (because of a lack of self-confidence in judgment or abilities rather than a lack of motivation or energy)

(5) goes to excessive lengths to obtain nurturance and support from others, to the point of volunteering to do things that are unpleasant

(6) feels uncomfortable or helpless when alone because of exaggerated fears of being unable to care for himself or herself

(7) urgently seeks another relationship as a source of care and support when a close relationship ends

(8) is unrealistically preoccupied with fears of being left to take care of himself or herself

---

*Reprinted with permission from the *Diagnostic and Statistical Manual of Mental Disorders, Fourth Edition*. Copyright 1994 American Psychiatric Association.

may be viewed as a compromise formation defending against hostility. Furthermore, dependent behavior can also be used to avoid reactivation of past traumatic experiences.

Biosocial Formulation

Millon and Everly (1985) speculate that dependent personalities exhibited fearful, withdrawing, or sad temperaments as infants. Accordingly, such behaviors were likely to elicit overly protective behavior from caretakers. Millon (1969) notes that these dependent individuals tend to have ectomorphic—thin and frail—or endomorphic—heavy and cumbersome—body types, which contribute to low energy thresholds and a lack of physical vigor.

Environmental factors such as parental overprotection, competitive deficits, and social-role programming appear to interact with these biological predispositions, resulting in the dependent personality pattern. Parental overprotection often precludes the development of autonomous coping behavior, such as assertiveness, problem solving, and decision making. Hend, Baker, and Williamson (1991) report that families of individuals with dependent personality disorders are characterized by low expressiveness and high control, as compared with families in clinical and normal control groups, which is indicative of the pervasive reinforcement of dependent behavior. Outside the parental relationship, these children often experience social humiliation and doubts about their efficacy in interpersonal situations. Through such repeated experiences, they learned, particularly as adolescents, that it is better to remain submissive than to strive to be competitive. Furthermore, cultural and social norms seem to reinforce passive dependent behavior patterns among women and endomorphically and ectomorphically built men. Finally, dependent personality patterns are self-perpetuating through reinforcement of dependent behaviors; avoidance of growth-promoting activities, that is, those that might be challenging, threatening, or anxiety producing; and self-detraction, by which they not only convince others that they are inferior, defective, and incapable of independence, but also themselves (Millon, 1981).

Cognitive-Behavioral Formulations

According to Beck et al. (1990), the dependent personality is rooted in basic assumptions about the self and the world. These individuals typically view themselves as helpless and inadequate, and the world as too dangerous for them to cope with alone. Accordingly, they conclude that they must rely on someone else who is stronger and more adequate to take care of and protect them. They must pay a considerable price for this security: (1) they must relinquish responsibility and subordinate their own needs; (2) they must relinquish opportunities to learn such skills as assertiveness, decision making, and problem solving; and (3) they must contend with fears of rejection and abandonment if their clinging relationship ends.

The main cognitive distortion of such dependent individuals is dichotomous thinking with respect to independence. For example, they believe that they are either totally connected to another and dependent or totally alone and independent, with no gradation between. Also, they believe that things are either "right" or "wrong," and that there is either "absolute success" or "absolute failure." Another cognitive distortion observed among dependent personalities is "catastrophizing," particularly regarding relationships. Common cognitive distortions are: "I never would be able to do that," "I can't," and "I'm too dumb to do that."

Turkat (1990) suggests a behavioral formulation for this disorder that centers on a pervasive fear of decision making and an inability to act assertively. Since these individuals have not previously learned either of these skills, these become basic therapeutic tasks, after their overwhelming anxiety is effectively managed.

Interpersonal Formulation

According to Benjamin (1993), persons with dependent personality disorder experienced sufficient caring and attention as infants to enable them to bond with others. They also learned to rely on others, and expect that others will be there to meet their needs. However, the parents of potential dependent-disordered individuals did not wean this level of nurturing when it was developmentally appropriate to do so. Subsequently, these individuals learned compliant dependent behavior, as well as to avoid autonomy at all costs. As a result, they developed poor self-concepts by default, and as adults continue to view themselves as inadequate and overly tolerant of the blaming of others. Because they have not learned to take care of self and life's demands, they must depend on others. Since they have limited coping resources, they must tolerate abuse, which is the price of the needed caretaking. Typically, dependent individuals-in-training were mocked by peers and siblings for their incompetence. As a result, their feelings of inadequacy and incompetence were reinforced and reconfirmed. In short, these individuals are characterized by marked submissiveness to a dominant other person, who presumably will provide unending nurturance and guidance. Such a relationship is maintained even if it means tolerating abuse, since dependent-disordered individuals believe themselves to be incompetent and unable to survive without the dominant other.

Integrative Formulation

The following integrative formulation provides a biopsychosocial explanation for how the dependent personality disorder develops and is maintained.

Biologically, these individuals are characterized by a low energy level. Their temperament is described as melancholic. As infants and young children, they were characterized as fearful, sad, or withdrawn. In terms of body types, they tend to have more ectomorphic or endomorphic builds (Millon, 1981).

Psychologically, dependent personality disorders can be understood and appreciated in terms of their view of themselves, their world view, and their life goal. The self view of these individuals tends to be a variant of the theme: "I'm nice, but inadequate (or fragile)." Their view of self is self-effacing, inept, and self-doubting. Their view of the world is some variant of the theme: "Others are here to take care of me, because I can't do it for myself." Their life goal is characterized by some variant of the theme: "Therefore, cling and rely on others at all cost."

The social features of this personality disorder can be described in terms of parental, familial, and environmental factors. The dependent personality is most likely to have been raised in a family in which parental overprotection was prominent. It is as if the parental injunction to the child was, "I can't trust you to do anything right (or well)." The dependent personality is likely to have been pampered and overprotected as a child. Contact with siblings and peers may engender feelings of unattractiveness, awkwardness, or competitive inadequacy, especially during the preadolescent and adolescent years. These can have a devastating impact on the individual, and further confirm his or her sense of self-deprecation and doubt. The dependent personality disorder becomes self-perpetuating through a process that involves a sense of self-doubt, an avoidance of competitive activ-

Table 5.3
Characteristics of Dependent Personality Disorder

1. Behavioral appearance	Docile, passive, nonassertive, lack of self-confidence
2. Interpersonal behavior	Pleasing; self-sacrificing; clinging, compliant; expect others to take responsibility
3. Cognitive style	Suggestible: Pollyannaish about interpersonal relations; overprotective—the "too good parent"
4. Feeling style	Pleasant, but anxious, timid, or sad when stressed
5. Parental injunction/ environmental factors	"You can't do it by yourself."
6. Biological/temperament	Low energy level; fearful, sad or withdrawn during infancy; melancholic
7. Self view	"I'm nice, but inadequate or fragile." Self-doubting
8. World view	"Others are here to take care of me" (because I can't do it myself)
9. Self and system perpetuant	Avoidance of competitive activities (+) dependence on others (+) self-deprecation→ reinforcement of dependent style

ity, and the availability of self-reliant individuals who are willing to take care of and make decisions for the dependent person in exchange for that person's self-sacrificing and docile friendship (Sperry & Mosak, 1993).

ASSESSMENT OF DEPENDENT PERSONALITY DISORDER

Several sources of information are useful in establishing a diagnosis and treatment plan for personality disorders. Observation, collateral information, and psychological testing are important adjuncts to the patient's self-report in the clinical interview. This section briefly describes some characteristic observations that the clinician makes and the nature of the rapport likely to develop in initial encounters with specific personality-disordered individuals. Characteristic response patterns on various objective (i.e., MMPI-2 and MCMI-II) and projective (i.e., Rorschach and TAT) tests are also described.

In the initial interview, individuals with dependent personality disorders will commonly wait for the clinician to initiate the conversation. After an opening statement by the clinician, these patients can present an adequate description of their current situation, but then will retreat to silence. Predictable comments are: "I don't know what to say. I've never seen a therapist before," or "Ask me questions so I'll know what's important to talk about." When the clinician responds and asks other questions, the cycle may repeat itself. Nonetheless, interviewing these individuals can be enjoyable, and establishing rapport is relatively easy. After some initial anxiety, they will begin to trust the clinician and the therapeutic process. So long as the clinician provides pleasant advice and support, and shows empathy for their indecisiveness and failures, the interview flows smoothly. However, when the clinician attempts to explore the detriments engendered by their submissiveness, they become uncomfortable and want support. If the dependency is not pursued with an empathic ear, they will change therapists. If pursued sympathetically, they will cooperate and meet their clinician's expectations. They answer questions to the point and will clarify and elaborate on demand. They can tolerate abrupt transitions and will allow deep feelings to be probed. But they cannot tolerate confrontation and interpretation of their dependency (Othmer & Othmer, 1989).

The Minnesota Multiphasic Personality Inventory (MMPI-2), the Millon Clinical Multiaxial Inventory (MCMI-II), the Rorschach Psychodiagnostic Test, and the Thematic Apperception Test (TAT) can be useful in diagnosing dependent personality disorder, as well as the dependent personality style or trait.

On the MMPI-2, the most likely profile is the 2-7/7-2 (Depression–Psychasthenia), which characterizes individuals who are passive, dependent, and docile. A high 3 (Hysteria) scale is common, as is a mildly elevated K (Correction) scale. Passivity and naiveté are reflected in a high L (Lie) scale, while the F (Frequency) scale is in the average range. Acceptance of the stereotypical female role is reflected by a low scale 5 (Masculinity–Femininity). Lack of resistance to coercion from authority shows in a low 4 (Psychopathic Deviate) scale. A low scale 9 (Hypomania) reflects passivity and lack of initiative (Meyer, 1993).

On the MCMI-II, a high score on scale 3 (Dependent) would be anticipated. An elevation on scale A (Anxiety) is common, particularly when these individuals feel insecure about placing their welfare in the hands of others (Choca et al., 1992).

With regard to the Rorschach, if dependent personalities feel accepted by the examiner and believe that the examiner expects a high number of responses, they will produce an extensive record. Otherwise, fewer than average responses can be expected. Most common are A (Animal), M (Human Movement), and P (Popular) responses. Finally, C (Color) tends to be used more often than F (Form) in determining responses (Meyer, 1993).

Generally speaking, the TAT responses of dependent personalities are not particularly distinctive. However, themes of dependency and compliance are common on card 2 (Bellak, 1993).

TREATMENT APPROACHES AND INTERVENTIONS

Treatment Considerations

The differential diagnoses for the dependent personality disorder include the histrionic personality disorder and the avoidant personality disorder. Common Axis I diagnoses that are associated with the dependent personality disorder include the anxiety disorders, particularly simple and social phobias, and panic disorders with or without agoraphobia. Other common DSM-III-R disorders include hypochondriasis, conversion disorders, and somatization disorders. The experience of losing a supportive person or relationship can lead to a number of affective disorders, including dysthymia and major depressive episodes. Finally, because persons with dependent personality disorders can have lifelong training in assuming the "sick role," they are especially prone to the factitious disorders.

In general, the long-range goal of psychotherapy with a dependent personality is to increase the individual's sense of independence and ability to function interdependently. At other times, the clinician may need to settle for a more modest goal—that is, helping the individual become a "healthier" dependent personality. Treatment strategies typically include challenging the individual's convictions or dysfunctional beliefs about personal inadequacy, and learning ways in which to increase assertiveness. A variety of treatment methods and modalities can be used to achieve these goals, as noted in the following section.

INDIVIDUAL PSYCHOTHERAPIES

For the various individual psychotherapeutic modalities, there are reports of successful treatment for dependent personality disorder. Although no large case series or controlled treatment trials have yet to be published, several case reports suggest that positive treatment outcomes are common. Treatment tends to be shorter and less difficult than for other personality disorders, such as the borderline, narcissistic or antisocial personality disorder.

Psychodynamic Psychotherapy Approach

A central purpose of psychodynamic psychotherapy is to help patients cope better with previous separations and object losses. Patients enter therapy with the unconscious wish to reinstate earlier relationships and bring them to a more satisfactory resolution. Accordingly, the clinician comes to symbolize the object losses, and therapy succeeds if the clinician becomes a better object than the objects of the patient's childhood. The clinician gratifies certain fundamental wishes that the parent-object did not adequately gratify, as well as provides a more reasonable and benign model for identification. If therapy is a success, the internalization of the objects will be more positive and less laden with anger and guilt, thereby making separation a genuine maturational event (Strupp & Binder, 1984). A major dilemma in the psychotherapy with patients with dependent personality disorders is that they do not readily relinquish the new object, and tend to cling tenaciously to the clinician.

In this form of resistance, the patient leans dependently on the clinician as an end in itself, rather than as a means to an end. Thus, as therapy unfolds, these patients may forget what complaint or symptom brought them into treatment, and their only purpose becomes the maintenance of their attachment to the clinician. Dreading termination, they tend to experience a reexacerbation of their initial symptoms. They will endeavor to make the clinician collude in their avoidance of making decisions or asserting themselves in the hope of continuing their dependency. The clinician, however, must frustrate these wishes and prompt independent thoughts and actions in these patients. By conveying that the anxiety produced by this frustration is tolerable and productive, the clinician encourages the patient toward achieving insight and independence (Gabbard, 1994).

In long-term psychodynamic psychotherapy, the emergence of a dependent transference toward the clinician is thus promoted, which is then dealt with in a way to promote emotional growth. Patients are told that extra sessions may be allowed early in therapy, particularly during periods of heightened anxieties. This assurance of readily available support aids in developing a trusting relationship with and transferring dependent wishes onto the clinician. The clinician must encourage patients to express feelings and wishes and to bear the anxiety of making decisions dealing with episodes of anxiety and accepting pleasurable experiences. Furthermore, the clinician will need to clarify and interpret the transference elements, as well as support the patients in finding more self-reliant ways of coping when they plead with the clinician to take a more directive role in their lives.

During the final stage of therapy, the clinician gradually increases the level of expectation for self-initiated behavior and autonomous decision making. The clinician reinforces the patient's increased ability to cope with crises without extra sessions and to self-soothe and self-manage episodes of heightened anxiety. This requires resolution of the patient's wish to be dependent and instead to accept a more self-reliant position in the therapeutic relationship (Hill, 1970). Finally, it should be noted that individuals with dependent personality disorders commonly create countertransference problems in their clinicians related to dependency conflicts. Thus clinicians must anticipate countertransference contempt or disdain toward dependent patients (Gabbard, 1994).

Time-Limited Dynamic Psychotherapy
Kantor (1992) notes that long-term analytic psychotherapy is arduous and time-consuming, and should be recommended primarily when patients are highly motivated and the dependency is ego syntonic. Otherwise, the treatment may become interminable because of such resistances as unwillingness to work hard in treatment because this means terminating therapy, which they anticipate will be unbearable. Generally speaking, long-term psychotherapy with motivated patients requires two to four sessions a week over three or more years to work through a dependent transference.

For these and other reasons, time-limited dynamic psychotherapy has been advocated as the treatment of choice for most of these patients (Flegenheimer, 1982; Gunderson, 1989). Knowing at the outset that treatment will end after 12, 16, or 20 sessions means that these patients must confront their deepest anxieties about loss and individuation, as well as their fantasies about unlimited nurturance and timelessness (Mann, 1973). Such time-limited therapies are most likely to succeed when three conditions are present: a circumscribed, dynamic conflict or focus; a patient who can quickly form a therapeutic alliance; and little or no tendency to act out or regress to severe dependency (Strupp & Binder, 1994; Luborsky, 1984). Time-limited therapy is less successful with dependent individuals who have limited ego strengths or greater degrees of separation anxiety (Gabbard, 1994). For such patients, Wallerstein (1986) suggests a supportive treatment approach in which sessions are tapered down to one every few months, provided there is no threat to termination.

Flegenheimer (1982) has critically reviewed six different brief dynamic psychotherapy approaches—those of Sifneos, Alexander, Mann, Malan, Davanloo, and Wolberg. He believes that Mann's, Alexander's, and Wolberg's approaches are tailor-made for the many dependent personality-disordered individuals. Passive, indecisive patients are likely to feel comfortable with the paternalistic stances of Alexander or Wolberg, where the clinician initially takes charge, gives advice, and makes decisions. The approach enables these patients to try new behaviors because they are "told to." The positive response to new behaviors engenders and reinforces those new patterns of behavior. Likewise, more passive dependent patients tend to do well with Mann's approach, wherein a termination date is set at the first session. The dependency of the patient allows the "golden glow" of Mann's first phase of therapy to develop to the fullest, setting the stage for subsequent disillusionment and preparing for a meaningful separation experience.

Mann's approach (1973) requires little modification of the standard analytically oriented approach, and requires the least amount of confrontation of the briefer psychotherapies. Not surprisingly, this rather gentle technique tends not to engender major resistances in dependent patients.

Time-limited approaches are advocated as the starting point for treatment of most dependent patients. For those who have multifocal conflicts or otherwise fail to improve in briefer therapies, longer term dynamic therapies, supportive therapy, or psychoanalysis would be treatment options.

Cognitive-Behavioral Approach

Beck et al. (1990) provide an extended description of the cognitive therapy approach with individuals with dependent personality disorders. The basic goal of therapy is increased autonomy and self-efficacy. Autonomy is defined as the capability to act independently of others, along with the capability to develop close and intimate relationships. Because dependent individuals are squeamish about the word "independent" and fear that competence will lead to abandonment, achieving these goals must be accomplished with considerable delicacy. Since these individuals often come to treatment anticipating that clinicians will solve their problems and make their decisions, it is necessary to allow some dependence initially in order to engage them. The structured collaborative nature of cognitive therapy encourages the dependent individual to play an active role in the treatment process, beginning with the agenda and goal setting. The use of guided discovery and Socratic questioning early in treatment helps these individuals to begin to face their own solutions and decisions, reducing overreliance on the therapist and others. As therapy proceeds, progress toward goals can be utilized as powerful evidence to challenge the dependent individual's assumptions of personal helplessness. Challenging the dichotomous belief about independence—that one is either totally dependent and helpless or totally independent and isolated—helps to modify the distorted notion that autonomy is a commitment to total alienation. Besides challenging and disputing automatic beliefs and maladaptive schemas concerning dependency and helplessness, therapists are encouraged to utilize behavioral methods such as assertiveness training and behavioral experiments, as well as to modify the very structure of therapy.

This modification can be accomplished in several ways, such as by gradually changing to a group format or concurrent individual and group therapy, "weaning" sessions by scheduling them less frequently toward the end of the therapy, or setting a specific termination date early in treatment and focusing therapy as preparation for termination. Since termination typically evokes rejection and abandonment schemas in these individuals, offering the option of one or two booster sessions—late in the course of treatment—following termination can ease the transition. In short, the cognitive treatment of dependent personality disorders begins with a collaborative relationship in which the therapist allows a measure of dependency, which is gradually replaced with guided discovery, and challenges the dichotomy beliefs of independence. As treatment proceeds, schema reconstruction and modification of the structure of treatment, along with behavioral methods, are utilized to achieve treatment goals.

A more behaviorally oriented approach to this disorder is based on the formulation that the dependent personality is hypersensitive to independent decision making (Turkat, 1990). The corresponding behavioral strategy is bidirectional anxiety management procedures focused on independent decision making. Since individuals with dependent personality disorder are often undersocialized, social skills training may be indicated. Assertive communication and friendship and dating skills are often minimal in lower functioning dependent patients. Fay and Lazarus (1993) offer cognitive-behavioral protocols in assertiveness, friendship, and dating skills.

Interpersonal Approach

For Benjamin (1993), psychotherapeutic interventions with persons with dependent personality disorders can be planned and evaluated in terms of whether they enhance collaboration, facilitate learning about maladaptive patterns and their roots, block these patterns, enhance the will to change, and effectively encourage new patterns.

Benjamin notes that the dependent individual's apparent attitude of friendly cooperation actually complicates the development of a collaborative therapeutic alliance. Essentially, eliciting more and better help from clinicians is the agenda for dependent individuals. They see no reason to collaborate with clinicians against their maladaptive pattern of dependency. The clinician's challenge at the onset of treatment is to engage with the position opposite their usual one: stop submitting, learn about being independent, and separate. Initially, this seems impossible for these individuals because, with their histories of intense enmeshment, they cannot understand what it means to be differentiated. They believe that there are only two options: to control others or to submit to others. Since they believe that controlling represents bossiness, aggressivity, and bullying of others, they reject it in favor of submission. However, if they are helped to understand that separation and competence, rather than control, are the opposite of submission, they can change. Blocking maladaptive patterns in dependent individuals often requires the assistance of their significant others, such as family members. The paradoxical suggestion that others restrict their offers of help at times when dependent individuals are functioning well is a way to reward independent behavior. Such suggestions must be followed with other interventions that change the strong wish to be dependent and strengthen the wish to become more competent and independent.

Essentially, dependent individuals must first recognize their dependent pattern and the high price they pay to maintain it, and then explore alternatives. To the extent that they can collaborate against "it" and face the present-day meaning of this pattern, they may decide to change. As this occurs, the implementation of a new pattern is relatively straightforward. Benjamin points out that standard behavioral techniques such as assertiveness communication and feeling identification and expression can be quite effective.

GROUP THERAPY

Group treatment has been shown to be successful in the treatment of dependent personality disorders. Two considerations are involved in deciding whether group treatment will be an effective format. The first consideration relates to the patient's degree of impairment; where motivation and potential for growth exist, a more interactional psychotherapy group may be indicated. Such a context provides a therapeutic milieu for exploring the inappropriateness of passive dependent behavior and for experimenting with greater assertiveness (Yalom, 1985). However, if dependent traits reflect severe personality impairment or the absence of prosocial behavior such as assertive communication, decision making, and negotiation, an ongoing supportive problem-solving group or a social skills training group might be indicated. The second consideration refers to whether referral should be made to a homogeneous group, with treatment targeted at dependency issues shared by all group members, or a heterogeneous group, where group members have different personality styles or disorders. Frances et al. (1984) provide selection criteria for both types of group formats. Clinical lore suggests that dependent patients tend to get "lost" in heterogeneous groups. Yalom (1985) seems to be describing the dependent personality in his discussion of the "silent patient" in groups. Yet time-limited assertiveness-training groups that are homogeneous and have clearly defined goals have been shown to be very effective (Lazarus, 1981).

Two studies involving the treatment of dependent patients have been reported in the literature. Montgomery (1971) utilized homogeneous group formats for dependent patients who were previously being seen in an individual format in a clinical setting. The patients were described as clinging and dependent, and as expecting magical cures and medication. Engagement within the group provided the patients with the opportunity to redirect their attention-seeking behavior from regressive to more socially adaptive purposes. Montgomery reports that all but three of 30 patients eventually discontinued medication. Sadoff and Collins (1968) reported group therapy for dependent patients who also stuttered. Weekly group treatment, which emphasized dynamic interpretation, was shown to be effective. Positive changes in stuttering and dependency were reported.

MARITAL/FAMILY THERAPY

The professional literature on family therapy interventions with the dependent personality disorders is almost nonexistent. Harbir (1981) notes that individuals with dependent personality disorders are usually brought to family therapy by their parents. They are frequently older adolescents or young adults between the ages of 20 and 35 who present with a neurotic or psychotic symptom. Harbir describes a prototypical case of a 29-year-old man with a diagnosis of dependent personality who essentially was totally dependent on his parents for his maintenance. A more functional younger sister had moved out on her own the previous year. Although he did some part-time work at home for his father, he neither made his own meals, cleaned his own room, nor washed his own clothes. He was content to live the rest of his life with his parents, if they would permit it. There was no clear-cut presenting problem, other than the identified patient's unwillingness to work outside the home. Clearly, the son, mother, and father were deeply enmeshed, although the son was much more dependent on the mother than the father, and vice versa. Structural techniques were employed by the clinician to decrease the intensity of the mother–child interaction. Essentially, various tasks were prescribed that encouraged the father and son to form a separate relationship. Tasks that encouraged social activities outside the family also were prescribed. Since the son had developed few peer relationships, these tasks initially were quite difficult for both the son and his parents.

After one year of family treatment, the son was able to emancipate sufficiently and could work and socialize outside the home. Could these results have been accomplished in individual therapy? Perhaps, but it was not likely in that time frame, and without some cooperation from the parents. Changing the enmeshed family relationship tends to be anxiety provoking for all parties, and thus there is considerable resistance from other family members when only one member of the family is in therapy.

Very little has been published on marital therapy with persons with dependent personality disorders. Malinow (1981) notes that dependent patients can function adequately if their marital partners consistently meet their needs, but typically become symptomatic and impaired when that support is withdrawn or withheld. Turkat (1990) believes that it is useful to engage the cooperation of the marital partner in treatment for two reasons: (1) because of the negative impact on the relationship as the dependent individual becomes less anxious and more independent, and (2) because the patient's progress can be facilitated if the partner collaborates in accomplishing the treatment goals. Barlow and Waddell (1985) describe a time-limited couples group for the treatment of agoraphobia. Most of the symptomatic partners exhibited features of the dependent personality. In group, the nonsymptomatic partners took the roles of "coach" and "confidant," collaborating on treatment goals. Taking on these roles meant relinquishing the role in which they reinforced their partner's agoraphobia and dependency. During the course of this 10-session treatment protocol, not only did panic and agoraphobia symptoms remit, but the marital relationship shifted from dependency to more interdependency.

MEDICATION

To date, the dependent personality disorder per se has not been subject to controlled pharmacological trials. Nevertheless, such individuals who present for treatment often exhibit Axis I diagnoses, particularly anxiety and depressive disorders. When appropriate, a concurrent anxiety or depressive disorder would be treated with a variety of psychotropic agents. Mavissakalian (1993) reviewed the indications for the use of psychotropic agents with the various anxiety disorders, as well as for combining cognitive-behavioral interventions with medication. Similarly, Rush and Hollon (1991) reviewed the indications for medication and cognitive-behavioral interventions for various depressive disorders.

However, if medication is not warranted for an Axis I disorder, caution should be exercised in considering medication for the Axis II dependent personality disorder. Anxiolytics are likely to be abused and antidepressants are inappropriate for reactive symptoms (Reid, 1989).

COMBINED/INTEGRATIVE TREATMENT APPROACHES

In many ways, the dependent personality is an "orphan" in the clinical literature, and this certainly is evident in the area of combined and integrative treatment. In the section on medication, reference was made to combined behavioral therapy for Axis I anxiety and depressive disorders concurrent with Axis II dependent personality disorder. The reader is referred to Mavissakalian (1993) and Rush and Hollon (1991) for excellent overviews of this literature.

Another type of combined treatment involves utilizing different modalities simultaneously. Barlow and Waddell's (1985) effort to combine behavior therapy in a group setting with couples was previously described. Not surprisingly, the results of combining modalities are noteworthy. Lazarus (1981, 1985) provides further documentation of the overall efficacy, and cost effectiveness, of multimodal interventions

Little has been written regarding integrative treatment. However, clinical practice is replete with efforts to utilize anxiety-reducing strategies in both dynamic and cognitive therapies.

Glantz and Goisman (1990) describe a unique integration of relaxation techniques with object-relations psychodynamic psychotherapy with dependent patients. A breath controlling and progressive muscle-relaxation strategy was used to merge split self-representations in the course of exploration psychotherapy. The technique was introduced after signs of split self-representation had been identified. Patients were taught the technique and it was prescribed as an intersession treatment task. Once they were able to relax adequately in session, they were asked for visual images of first one and then another of the conflicting self-representations. After clear images had been elicited and discussed, they were encouraged to merge the images. Twenty-four of the 27 personality-disordered patients in the study, many of whom were dependent personalities, responded with greater compliance, improved interpersonal relationships, and reduced resistance.

Handler (1989) reports integrating Ericksonian hypnotic methods with psychodynamically oriented psychotherapy in the treatment of a woman diagnosed with dependent personality disorder and somatoform disorder. The results were positive and were sustained over a two-year period.

CHAPTER 6

Histrionic Personality Disorder

The histrionic personality disorder has a long history, dating back to some 4,000 years ago, when it was called "hysteria" (Veith, 1977). The modern roots of the histrionic personality are traceable to Freud's description of cases of "hysterical neurosis," which today would be classified as a type of somatoform disorder. DSM-I had no category for hysterical personality, although some of its traits were encompassed by the diagnostic category "emotionally unstable personality." DSM-II listed hysterical personality with "histrionic personality disorder" in parentheses. In DSM-III, it was designated as histrionic personality disorder, and because of its considerable overlap with borderline personality disorder, several changes were made in the criteria in DSM-III-R (Pfohl, 1991). Now DSM-IV has further modified the criteria to better distinguish histrionic from borderline. Nonetheless, psychodynamically oriented clinicians remain dissatisfied, as the new criteria do not allow for the more highly functioning patient. Thus psychoanalytic writers prefer to use the designation hysterical personality disorder for higher functioning individuals and histrionic personality disorder for more primitive, lower functioning individuals who clearly meet DSM-IV criteria (Gabbard, 1994). The disorder appears to be more common in women than in men. Prevalence rates are estimated to be 2 to 3 percent in the general population and 10 to 15 percent in clinical settings.

This chapter describes the characteristic features of the histrionic personality disorder and its related style. Five clinical formulations of the disorder and psychological assessment indicators are highlighted. A variety of treatment approaches, modalities, and intervention strategies are also described.

CHARACTERISTICS OF THE HISTRIONIC PERSONALITY STYLE AND DISORDER

The histrionic personality can be thought of as spanning a continuum from healthy to pathological, with the histrionic personality style at the healthy end and the histrionic personality disorder at the pathological end. Table 6.1 compares and contrasts the histrionic personality style and disorder.

The clinical presentation of the histrionic personality disorder can be characterized by the following behavioral, interpersonal, cognitive, and emotional styles.

The behavioral style is charming, dramatic, and expressive, while also being demanding, self-indulgent, and inconsiderate. Persistent attention seeking, mood lability, capriciousness, and superficiality further characterize this behavior.

Interpersonally, these individuals tend to be exhibitionistic and flirtatious in their manner, with attention seeking and manipulativeness being prominent. They also tend to have empathic deficits, just as do those with narcissistic personality disorders.

The cognitive or thinking style of this personality can be characterized as impulsive and thematic, rather than analytical, precise, and field independent. Their tendency is to be nonanalytic, vague, and field dependent. They are highly suggestible and rely heavily on hunches and intuition. They avoid awareness of their own hidden dependency and other self-knowledge, and tend to be "other directed" with respect to the need for approval from others. Therefore, they can easily dissociate their "real" or inner selves from their "public" or outer selves.

Their emotional or feeling style is characterized by exaggerated emotional displays and excitability, including irrational outbursts and temper tantrums. Although they are constantly seeking reassurance that they are loved, they respond with only superficial warmth and charm and are generally emotionally shallow. Finally, they are exquisitely sensitive to rejection.

The following two case examples further illustrate differences between the histrionic personality disorder (Ms. P.) and the histrionic personality style (Mr. M.).

Table 6.1
Comparison of the Histrionic Personality Style and Disorder

Personality Style	Personality Disorder
• Enjoy compliments and praise.	• Constantly seek or demand reassurance, approval, or praise.
• Charming, engaging, and appropriately seductive in appearance and behavior.	• Inappropriately sexually seductive in appearance and behavior.
• Attentive to their appearance and grooming, enjoying clothes, style, and fashion.	• Overly concerned with physical attractiveness.
• Lively and fun-loving, often impulsive, but can delay gratification.	• Express emotion with inappropriate exaggeration; self-centered and little tolerance for gratification.
• Enjoy being the center of attention, and can rise to the occasion when all eyes are on them.	• Uncomfortable in situations where they cannot be the center of attention.
• Sensation oriented, emotionally demonstrative, and physically affectionate. React emotionally, but appropriately.	• Display rapidly shifting and shallow expression of emotion.
• Utilize a style of speech that is appropriately global and specific.	• Utilize a style of speech that is excessively impressionistic and lacking in detail.

Case Study: Histrionic Personality Disorder

Ms. P. is a 20-year-old undergraduate student who requested psychological counseling at the College Health Services for "boyfriend problems." She actually had taken a nonlethal overdose of minor tranquilizers the previous day in an attempt, she said, to kill herself because "life wasn't worth living" after her boyfriend had left the afternoon before. An attractive woman, she was well dressed and wore makeup and nail polish, which contrasted sharply with the very casual appearance of most women on campus. During the initial interview, she was warm and charming, maintained good eye contract, and was mildly seductive. At two points in the interview, she was emotionally labile, shifting from smiling elation to tearful sadness. Her boyfriend had accompanied her to the evaluation session and asked to talk to the clinician. He stated that he had left the patient because she made demands on him that he could not meet, and that he "hadn't been able to satisfy her emotionally or sexually." Also, he noted that he could not afford to "take her out every night and party."

Case Study: Histrionic Personality Style

Mr. M. is a 41-year-old literary agent who spent the early years of his career representing nonfiction writers with major publishing houses. He has been quite successful for several years, but also has become somewhat disenchanted with his behind-the-scenes efforts. He had made several of his clients extraordinarily wealthy and famous, but dreamed of the time when he, too, would be financially independent and in the limelight. When cable TV licenses became available, he saw the opportunity to fulfill his dream. He would become president of his own station and host his own talk show, as he had several high visibility clients whom he could persuade to be guests. He set out to garner financing for his plan. With his charming manner and enticing vision, he soon intrigued several backers and got the station launched. The problem was that he had not thought much about the production side of the enterprise, and he quickly arranged for interviews for an executive producer. William T. was the fourth person he interviewed, and Mr. M. knew as soon as he walked in that he was right for the job. After a 10-minute interview, William was hired. Mr. M.'s hunches about William and the success of the talk show proved to be right.

DSM-IV Description and Criteria

Table 6.2 presents the DSM-IV description and criteria.

FORMULATIONS OF HISTRIONIC PERSONALITY DISORDER

Psychodynamic Formulations

Gabbard (1990) argues that the histrionic personality disorder needs to be distinguished from the hysterical personality disorder. The latter has a central place in the tradition of psychoanalytic thinking and refers to a group of patients who are higher functioning and healthier than those in the group characterized by DSM-IV criteria. Female histrionics typically lack maternal nurturance and turn to their fathers for gratification of their dependence needs. They learn that they can gain the father's attention by flirtation and exhibitionistic displays of emotion. As they mature, they learn that they must repress their genital sexuality to remain "Daddy's little girl." Similarly, histrionic males will have also experienced maternal deprivation and turned to their fathers for nurturance. If the father is emotionally

Table 6.2
DSM-IV Description and Criteria for Histrionic Personality Disorder*

301.50 Histrionic Personality Disorder

A pervasive pattern of excessive emotionality and attention seeking, beginning by early adulthood and present in a variety of contexts, as indicated by five (or more) of the following:

(1) is uncomfortable in situations in which he or she is not the center of attention

(2) interaction with others is often characterized by inappropriate sexually seductive or provocative behavior

(3) displays rapidly shifting and shallow expression of emotions

(4) consistently uses physical appearance to draw attention to self

(5) has a style of speech that is excessively impressionistic and lacking in detail

(6) shows self-dramatization, theatricality, and exaggerated expression of emotion

(7) is suggestible, i.e., easily influenced by others or circumstances

(8) considers relationships to be more intimate than they actually are

*Reprinted with permission from the *Diagnostic and Statistical Manual of Mental Disorders, Fourth Edition*. Copyright 1994 American Psychiatric Association.

unavailable, they may develop either a passive, effeminate identification, or a hypermasculine one in reaction to their anxiety about effeminacy. These men may not become homosexuals, but their heterosexual relationships are means of reassuring themselves with regard to underlying genital inadequacy. They will be disappointed with all women as they cannot measure up to their mothers. Some will choose a celibate lifestyle in order to maintain their loyalty to their mothers, whereas others will indulge in macho behavior such as body building and Don Juanism (i.e., compulsive seduction of women) to reassure themselves that they are "real men" (Kellerman & Burry, 1989).

Biosocial Formulation

Millon (1981) and Millon and Everly (1985) note that individuals with histrionic personality disorders often display a high degree of emotional lability and responsiveness during infancy and early childhood, and they attribute this to low excitability thresholds for limbic and posterior hypothalamic nuclei. However, environmental factors seem to play the major role in the development of this pathology. Millon and Everly (1985) list three such factors: parental reinforcement of attention-seeking behavior, histrionic parental role models, and reinforcement of interpersonally manipulative behavior. In effect, as children, these individuals learned to employ cuteness, charm, attractiveness, and seduction to secure parental reinforcement. Furthermore, this disorder is self-perpetuated through short-lived relationships, preoccupation with externals, and massive repression. Specifically, by sealing off and repressing aspects of their inner worlds, histrionic individuals deny themselves opportunities to develop psychologically.

Cognitive-Behavioral Formulations

Beck et al. (1990) describe a cognitive therapy view of the histrionic personality disorder based on specific underlying assumptions and cognitive distortions. Two underlying assumptions are posited: "I am inadequate and unable to handle life by myself," and "I must be loved by everyone to be worthwhile." Believing that they are incapable of caring for themselves, histrionic individuals actively seek the attention and approval of others and expect others to take care of them and their needs. The belief that they must be loved and approved by others promotes rejection sensitivity. Finally, feeling inadequate and desperate for approval, they are under considerable pressure to seek attention by "performing" for others. These beliefs also give rise to a thinking style characterized as impressionistic, global, and unfocused, which is not conducive to a differentiated sense of self. Not surprisingly, this global, exaggerated thinking style engenders common cognitive distortions (Beck, 1967), such as dichotomous thinking, overgeneralization, and emotional reasoning.

Taking a more behavioral tack, Turkat (1990) categorizes the histrionic personality disorder into two types: the controlling type, in which the basic motivation is achieving total control through the use of manipulative and dramatic ploys; and the reactive type, in which the basic motivation is seeking reassurance and approval. Turkat does not believe that the controlling type is amenable to behavior treatment. Unable to read others' emotions and interventions accurately, these individuals remain shallow, self-centered, and uncomfortable when immediate reinforcement is not immediately forthcoming from others. In short, they suffer from a primary deficit in empathy.

Interpersonal Formulation

For Benjamin (1993), persons with histrionic personality disorders are likely to be loved for their good looks and entertainment value, rather than for competence or personal strength. They have learned that physical appearance and charm can be used to control important others. The households of histrionic personalities tended to be shifting stages. Unpredictable changes stemmed from parental instability, possibly associated with alcohol or substance use. The chaos in these families was more likely to be dramatic and interesting than primitive and life threatening, as with borderline personalities. The help-seeking histrionic subtypes were likely to be nurtured for being ill. They learned that complaints and disabilities were an effective way to elicit warm concern. Along with encouragement of denial, these families rewarded sickness. Finally, they exhibit a strange fear of being ignored, together with a wish to be loved and taken care of by important others, who can be controlled through charm or sickness. In short, a friendly trust is accompanied by a secretly disrespectful agenda of forcing delivery of the desired nurturance and love. Inappropriate seductive behaviors and manipulative suicide attempts exemplify such coercions.

Integrative Formulation

The following integrative formulation may be helpful in understanding how the histrionic personality disorder develops and is maintained.

Biologically and temperamentally, the histrionic personality disorder appears to be quite different from the dependent personality disorder. Unlike the dependent personality, the histrionic personality is characterized by a high energy level and emotional and autonomic reactivity. Millon and Everly (1985) noted that histrionic adults tended to display a high degree of emotional lability and responsiveness in their infancy and early childhood. Their temperaments then can be characterized as hyperresponsive and externally oriented for gratification.

Psychologically, histrionic personality disorder has the characteristic view of self, world view, and life goal. The self view of the histrionic will be some variant of the theme: "I am sensitive and everyone should admire and approve of me." The world view will be some variant of: "Life makes me nervous, so I am entitled to special care and consideration." Their life goals are some variant of the theme: "Therefore, play to the audience and have fun, fun, fun." It should be noted that although there are expectations of special entitlement in the histrionic personality, these expectations are somewhat different than in the narcissistic personality disorder. Both are sensitive to minor slights and are easily angered when ignored. However, these slights tend to be easily attenuated in the histrionic, as the deflection of self-esteem involves only a threat to dependency, whereas for the narcissist, these slights are a threat to the integrity of the self. Thus the narcissist is more likely to employ splitting, projective identification, and other primitive defenses than is the histrionic (Kellerman & Burry, 1989).

In addition to biological and psychological factors, social factors, such as parenting style and injunction and family and environmental factors, influence the development of the histrionic personality. The parental injunction for the histrionic personality involves reciprocity: "I'll give you attention, if you do X." A parenting style that employs minimal or inconsistent discipline helps to reinforce the histrionic pattern. The histrionic child is likely to grow up with at least one manipulative or histrionic parent who reinforces the child's histrionic and attention-seeking behavior. Finally, the following sequence of self and system perpetuants are likely to be seen in the histrionic personality disorder: denial of one's real or inner self; a preoccupation with externals; the need for excitement and attention seeking, which leads to a superficial charm and interpersonal presence; and the need for external approval. This, in turn, further reinforces the dissociation and denial of the real or inner self from the public self, and the cycle continues (Sperry & Mosak, 1993).

Table 6.3
Characteristics of Histrionic Personality Disorder

1.	Behavioral appearance	Charming/excitement seeking; labile, capricious, superficial
2.	Interpersonal behavior	Attention getting/manipulative; exhibitionistic/flirtatious
3.	Cognitive style	Impulsive, thematic, field-dependent; avoid awareness of hidden dependencies
4.	Feeling style	Exaggerated emotional display
5.	Parental injunction/ environmental factors	"I'll give you attention when you do what I want." Manipulative/histrionic parental role models: minimal or inconsistent disciplining
6.	Biological/temperament	Hyperresponsive infantile pattern, externally oriented for gratification
7.	Self view	"I need to be noticed"; externally oriented for gratification
8.	World view	"Life makes me so nervous, so I'm entitled to special care and consideration."
9.	Self and system perpetuant	Preoccupation with externals (+) repression→ denial of shadow and inner life→ reinforcement of need for approval and histrionic style

ASSESSMENT OF HISTRIONIC PERSONALITY DISORDER

Several sources of information are useful in establishing a diagnosis and treatment plan for personality disorders. Observation, collateral information, and psychological testing are important adjuncts to the patient's self-report in the clinical interview. This section briefly describes some characteristic observations that the clinician makes and the nature of the rapport likely to develop in initial encounters with specific personality-disordered individuals. Characteristic response patterns on various objective (i.e., MMPI-2 and MCMI-II) and projective (i.e., Rorschach and TAT) tests are also described.

Interviewing individuals with histrionic personality disorders can be enjoyable but challenging. Initially, they may be more interested in admiration and approval than in a therapeutic relationship. Rapport, therefore, may be difficult to establish. Exaggerated emotionality, vagueness, superficiality, and phoniness are common in the first encounter. With a male clinician, histrionic women may be flirtatious and seductive, whereas with a female clinician, they are more likely to engage in a power struggle. To elicit sufficient information to complete a diagnostic evaluation usually requires the clinician to overcome their vagueness and dramatic exaggerations. Open-ended and unstructured questions are not useful, as these individuals easily become sidetracked. It is preferable to pursue a main theme such as a work problem or an interpersonal conflict and elicit concrete examples, while curbing rambling and contradictions. Confronting contradictions typically results in anger and loss of rapport. Instead, the clinician should express empathy and encouragement. It is predictable that when they feel that empathy and understanding are slipping away, they will return to dramatization (Othmer & Othmer, 1989).

The Minnesota Multiphasic Personality Inventory (MMPI-2), the Millon Clinical Multiaxial Inventory (MCMI-II), the Rorschach Psychodiagnostic Test, and the Thematic Apperception Test (TAT) can be useful in diagnosing histrionic personality disorder, as well as the histrionic personality style or trait.

On the MMPI-2, the 2-3/3-2 (Depression–Hysteria) profile is most commonly found. When clinically distressed, these individuals are likely to have elevations on 2 greater than 70. If not, scale 3 will be more elevated. The 3-4/4-3 (Hysteria–Psychopathic Deviant) and 4-9/9-4 (Psychopathic Deviant–Hypermania) patterns are also noted in these individuals (Graham, 1990). Scales 4, 7 (Psychasthenia), and 8 (Schizophrenia) may also be moderately elevated, with scale 4 reflecting their tendency to be overdramatic and self-absorbed, self-doubt and anxiety raising the 7 score, and impulsive emotionality elevating the 8. Scale 5 is also likely to be elevated in men, but quite low in women, reflecting the association of hysteria with traditional feminine role behavior (Meyer, 1993).

On the MCMI-II, elevations on scale 4 (Histrionic) are expected. Because these individuals are attention seekers, scales 1 (Schizoid) and 2 (Avoidant) tend to be very low, whereas H (Somatization) may be high, as somatization can be used as an attention-getting device, as can N (Bipolar–Manic) (Choca et al., 1992).

On the Rorschach, these individuals provide a low number of responses, as well as a low number of W (Whole), M (Human Movement), C (Pure Color), and shading (Y, YF, or T) responses. Occasionally, they will give a "blood" response to a color card.

On the TAT, these individuals typically produce stories containing dependency and control themes. Their stories may also become personalized, generating some affective display. Occasionally, blocking occurs on cards with sexual or aggressive percepts. Rarely, primitive splitting may be noted in characters that are all good or all bad on incongruous juxtapositions (Bellak, 1993).

TREATMENT APPROACHES AND INTERVENTIONS

Treatment Considerations

The differential diagnosis of the histrionic personality disorder includes the narcissistic personality disorder and the dependent personality disorder. In addition, Axis II combines the histrionic borderline disorder, which is a decompensated version of the histrionic personality disorder. Associated DSM-IV Axis I diagnoses are, in order of occurrence: dysthymia; acute anxiety syndromes, such as simple and social phobias; and the somatoform disorders, particularly conversion reactions and hypochondriasis. Other disorders are the obsessive-compulsive disorder and the dissociative disorders, particularly fugue states. Finally, major depression and bipolar disorders are common in the decompensated histrionic personality disorder.

The treatment of the histrionic personality disorder may present a considerable challenge to the clinician. General treatment goals include helping the individual to integrate gentleness with strength, moderating emotional expression, and encouraging warmth, genuineness, and empathy. Because the histrionic personality can present as dramatic, impulsive, seductive, and manipulative, with the potential for suicidal gestures, the clinician needs to discuss the matter of limits early in the course of therapy regarding professional boundaries and personal responsibilities.

INDIVIDUAL PSYCHOTHERAPY APPROACHES

This section briefly reviews the major psychotherapeutic approaches for treating the histrionic personality disorder in an individual psychotherapy format. Later sections will describe other treatment formats, such as group therapy, couples therapy, and pharmacotherapy. The individual treatment approaches are the psychoanalytic, cognitive-behavioral, and interpersonal.

Psychodynamic Psychotherapy Approach

Gabbard (1990) is quite optimistic about the responsiveness of higher functioning individuals with histrionic personality disorders to psychoanalytically oriented psychotherapy. He reports that such individuals readily develop a therapeutic alliance and perceive the therapist as helpful. He further believes that with lower functioning individuals with this personality disorder, treatment should employ therapeutic strategies utilized for the borderline personality disorder.

Winer and Pollock (1989) indicate that the basic dynamic in all presentations of the histrionic personality disorder is the excessive, unresolved effort to have all of their needs met by someone else. The general goal of dynamically oriented therapies is to examine the origins of the pattern and explore the neurotic strategies—seductiveness, temper tantrums, charm, or logical thinking—that these individuals employ in order to fulfill their needs.

The classical psychoanalytic method emphasizes therapist neutrality and requires that the patient have sufficient ego strength to regress in a controlled manner. The transference that develops is analyzed with mutative interpretations, and presumably leads to enduring personality change. Thus proper handling of transference, particularly erotic transference, is important. Gabbard (1990) notes that the mishandling of erotic transference is probably the most frequent cause of treatment failure with these patients. Particularly with those who are more disturbed and unstable, transference distortions require that resolving transference distortions by interpretation be undertaken with great caution. In fact, some (Khan, 1975; Havens, 1976) suggest that erotic transference not be allowed to develop too firmly or be interpreted. Rather, counterprojective techniques are advised. These are direct or subtle, verbal or nonverbal responses that communicate to the patient that the therapist is not a transference figure of childhood (Havens, 1976).

Brief Dynamic Psychotherapy

Although long-term psychoanalytically oriented psychotherapy is considered the mainstay of dynamic treatment (Quality Assurance Project, 1991), time-limited individual psychotherapy may also be quite useful, particularly with higher functioning histrionic individuals. The approaches of Malan (1976) and Sifneos (1972, 1984) seem quite promising. The short-term anxiety-provoking psychotherapy (STAPP) approach developed by Sifneos may be a particularly "good fit" for highly functioning histrionic individuals who present with satisfactory impersonal relationships, psychological mindedness, the ability easily to engage and interact with a therapist, and a circumscribed presenting complaint. On the other hand, Mann's (1973, 1984) time-limited approach, which requires patients to engage and disengage from therapy quickly "without suffering unduly," may pose considerable difficulty for these individuals, who characteristically develop intense and sticky transferences with therapists (Chodoff, 1989). Winston and Pollack (1991) describe brief adaptive psychotherapy (BAP) as particularly effective with histrionic individuals. BAP has an ego psychological orientation that focuses on maladaptive patterns of beliefs and behaviors. The maladaptive pattern is thoroughly assessed as its underlying elements are explored in detail, with particular attention to transference and resistance.

Cognitive-Behavioral Approach

According to Beck et al. (1990), cognitive therapy is particularly appropriate for treating patients with histrionic personality disorders, provided they remain in treatment. Although usually cooperative and motivated for therapy, the histrionic's global, diffuse thinking style is quite different from the systematic, structural nature of cognitive therapy. Thus they initially find treatment difficult and frustrating as they learn to focus attention on a single issue at a time, and then to monitor their thoughts and feelings. A number of conditions are necessary for cognitive treatment of this disorder to be successful. Since these individuals are generally dependent and demanding in relationships, the use of collaborative and guided discovery is particularly applicable. Taking an active role and utilizing questioning are quite helpful in stemming the histrionic individual's view of clinicians as rescuers and saviors. Setting limits that are clear and firm, while rewarding assertive requests within these limits and demonstrating caring in other ways, is another necessary condition of treatment. The next condition is establishing treatment goals, which must be meaningful and be perceived as urgent by these patients, and be specific and concrete enough that short-term, as well as long-term, benefits can become realities. This counters the histrionic individual's tendency to set broad, vague, noble-sounding goals. An important key to keeping these people in therapy is achieving one or more of the specific, short-term goals that were collaboratively established.

The mainstay of treatment involves the challenging of automatic thoughts; the self-monitoring of cognition, which is helpful in controlling impulsivity; and the restructuring, modification, and interpretation of maladaptive schemas. Challenging the most basic assumptions, such as "I am inadequate and have to rely on others to survive," is aided by cognitive-behavioral methods, such as assertion, problem solving, and behavioral experiments, which can increase these patients' self-efficacy and help them feel more competent. Another central belief that must be modified is that the loss of a relationship is always disastrous. Fantasizing about the reality of what would happen if a relationship were to end, and recalling how they survived before that relationship began, can help these individuals "decatastrophize" their beliefs about rejection. The behavioral approach has not been shown to be effective with the controlling type of histrionic personality (Turkat & Maisto, 1985; Turkat, 1990). The reactive type is more amenable to change, specifically with empathy training. Turkat (1990) describes this intervention, which consists of social skills training in active listening, paraphrasing, and reflection. The goal is to teach these patients to focus increasingly on the needs and feelings of other people. Role playing with video feedback has been especially effective. The use of dramatic behavioral experiments and training in problem-solving skills are also advocated by Beck et al. (1990).

In short, an effective cognitive therapy approach to the histrionic personality disorder will be systematic and structural (including firm limit setting and specific treatment goals) and will include cognitive (disputation of automatic thoughts and schemas and restructuring of basic maladaptive beliefs and schemas) as well as behavioral methods.

Interpersonal Approach

For Benjamin (1993), psychotherapeutic interventions with persons with histrionic personality disorders can be planned and evaluated in terms of whether they enhance collaboration, facilitate learning about maladaptive patterns and their roots, block these patterns, enhance the will to change, and effectively encourage new patterns.

Benjamin notes that the establishment of a therapeutic alliance facilitating collaboration with the histrionic individual must be based on a knowledge of the basic pattern, wishes, and fears of that individual. It is essential that the therapist communicate warmth and competent support, while not reinforcing the histrionic's dependent, needy position. The working contract is with the individual's observing ego, whereas the "enemy" is the damaging pattern. A major task in beginning treatment is to transform the histrionic's view of treatment from a way of making fantasies come true to a place where personal development can be facilitated.

The task of learning to recognize patterns is complicated in that histrionic individuals have not sufficiently developed an observing ego to help them to recognize and reflect on patterns. In fact, they have come to believe that if they were to become competent, they would be left alone and no one would care for them. Whereas the female histrionic can internalize the female clinician's modeling of a benign and constructive examination of patterns, the male clinician must help the individual confront her fears that if she becomes competent, the clinician will decide that she is unattractive and will stop treatment.

Next, the clinician focuses the histrionic individual's attention on potentially destructive patterns of acting out based on underlying fears and wishes. By providing gentle challenges, the clinician protects these patients from their own past. The goal is to expand options and enhance awareness in light of what is being learned about patterns. The therapist does not block patterns with advice giving, but reviews options. Developing the will to change patterns is enhanced if these patterns can be uncovered and clearly connected in an experiential way to the past. This often facilitates the individual's "decision" to give up the goals that drive the patterns. Finally, Benjamin advocates utilizing traditional techniques from other approaches to build new patterns and ways of functioning, once the "unconscious underbrush" has been cleared away.

GROUP THERAPY

The literature on the histrionic personality is quite interesting with regard to the treatability of this disorder in group settings. There are clear warnings in the older psychoanalytic literature about the effect of these patients on other group members. Slavson (1939) cautioned that their changeability and unpredictability would engender stress and anxiety in a group, and advocated that these patients be treated only in individual therapy. Conversely, contemporary clinicians such as Gabbard (1990, 1994) contend that histrionic patients who are appropriate for individual dynamic psychotherapy are also appropriate for dynamic group psychotherapy. In fact, Gabbard finds that these patients are highly valued by other group members for their ability to express affects directly, and because of their concern for these other members.

The group treatment format has a number of advantages over individual treatment. First, a group setting frustrates the wishes and demands these patients have for the exclusive attention of the therapist, and so challenges the approval-seeking posture of these patients. Thus the risk that an eroticized transference will develop is relatively small as compared with individual therapy.

Second, their global cognitive style and associated defenses of repression and denial can be more effectively treated in a group setting. Group members will confront the distorted manner in which histrionic patients view themselves and others, including their style, omission of details, and focus on affects over thoughts.

Finally, histrionic patients tend to form positive maternal transferences, and they expect the group to make up for the maternal nurturance they missed as children (Gabbard, 1990). Whereas this transference is challenging for the clinician in individual therapy, it is considerably "diluted" in a group treatment format.

Relatively little has been published about the effectiveness of group treatment of histrionic patients, but one study is encouraging. Cass, Silvers, and Abrams (1972) reported a case in which behavioral group treatment significantly modified inappropriate passivity, manipulativeness, and acting out, which were replaced by more effective assertive interpersonal behavior.

The question of indications and contraindications has been addressed by some writers. Halleck (1978) cautions that histrionic patients who cannot participate in a group process without monopolizing or disrupting it should be excluded. Gabbard (1990), however, points out that histrionic individuals might still be candidates for group therapy if they are concurrently in individual psychotherapy. Sheidlinger and Porter (1980) indicate that combined treatment—individual plus group therapy—may be the treatment of choice for such patients.

MARITAL/FAMILY THERAPY

Although there are no reports of family therapy per se with histrionic patients, there are a number of case reports on marital therapy with these patients. Typically, the couple consists of an obsessive-compulsive husband and a histrionic wife, with the obsessive-compulsive spouse tending to assume increasing responsibility while the histrionic spouse becomes increasingly helpless (Berman, 1983). Treatment may be sought following some primitive outburst, which can include a threat of self-destructive behavior, typically during separation or divorce. The loss of a stable dependent figure is a major stressor for the histrionic patient, who may exhibit aggressive attention-seeking behavior, increased affective display and seductiveness, and possibly promiscuity in an effort to make the other spouse jealous, and so on (Harbir, 1981).

The general goal of treatment is to facilitate changing this pattern in both spouses, which is accomplished better in a couples format than in individual sessions. Harbir (1981) offers a treatment protocol for couples where divorce and child custody are issues.

MEDICATION

Drug trials on histrionic personality disorder per se have not been reported. Nor are such trials likely. However, from a target symptom or dimensional (i.e., trait cluster) perspective, there are promising indications for the effective utilization of psychotropics in the treatment of certain histrionic personalities.

The most obvious indications for medication are when concurrent Axis I presentations are noted. When severe depression is the presenting symptom, antidepressants are probably indicated. The choice of cyclic or serotonergic blockers is made on the basis of specific depressive features and the side-effects profile.

When the presentation involves exquisite rejection sensitivity, craving for attention, demanding behavior, hyperphagia, and hypersomnia when depressed, the depressive subtype of hysteroid dysphoria may exist (Liebowitz & Klein, 1981). Monoamine oxidase inhibitors (MAOIs) have been found to be the medication of choice.

When no obvious Axis I presentation is appreciated, but dimensional cluster symptoms are noted (i.e., affective constability, compulsivity, or cognitive-perceptual disorganization), specific agents may be indicated (Siever & Davis, 1991). Lower functioning histrionic patients are characterized by affective instability and some impulsivity. Sertraline, a serotonergic blocker, has demonstrated some efficacy with such patients (Kavoussi et al., 1994).

INTEGRATED AND COMBINED TREATMENT APPROACH

The basic premise of this book is that symptomatic and lower functioning personality-disordered individuals are less likely to respond to a single-treatment approach or modality. Since personality disorders are biopsychosocial phenomena (Pies, 1992), combined or integrative, tailored treatment is indicated, particularly for the more symptomatic and severe presentations. Stone (1992) advocates combined treatments, wherein two or more approaches or modalities are utilized concurrently or in tandem.

Previously, it was mentioned that combining individual psychotherapy with concurrent group therapy was indicated for histrionic patients who monopolized or were disruptive in group settings (Sheidlinger & Porter, 1980). It has also been noted that behavioral techniques may be integrated with a psychodynamic or cognitive approach. Finally, medications may be a useful adjunct to psychotherapy, either concurrently or in tandem, if specific Axis I or Axis II symptoms or trait clusters are prominent.

CHAPTER 7

Narcissistic Personality Disorder

The narcissistic personality disorder has been the subject of widespread interest among mental health professionals. Prior to DSM-III, this disorder was not included in DSMs or in the International Classification of Disorders (ICD). The narcissistic personality has been dubbed one of the neurotic personalities of our times (Sperry, 1991b). The widespread use of the term narcissistic personality by psychodynamically oriented clinicians was a major impetus for the inclusion of the disorder into DSM-III (Gunderson, Ronningstam, & Smith, 1991).

Prevalence estimates of this disorder in the general population are less than 1 percent. In clinical populations, the range is between 2 and 16 percent. However, the number of individuals exhibiting significant narcissistic traits is very large (Stone, 1993).

This chapter describes the characteristic features of this disorder and its related personality style, five different clinical formulations, psychological assessment indicators, and a variety of treatment approaches and intervention strategies.

CHARACTERISTICS OF THE NARCISSISTIC PERSONALITY STYLE AND DISORDERS

The narcissistic personality is quite common in Western culture, particularly among those in certain occupations and professions, such as law, medicine, entertainment, sports, and politics. It can be thought of as spanning a continuum from healthy to the pathological, with the narcissistic personality style at the healthy end and the personality disorder at the pathological end. Table 7.1 compares and contrasts differences between the narcissistic style and disorder.

Narcissistic personality disorder is characterized by the following behavioral and interpersonal, cognitive, and affective styles.

Behaviorally, narcissistic individuals are seen as conceited, boastful, and snobbish. They appear self-assured and self-centered, and they tend to dominate conversations, to seek admiration, and to act in a pompous and exhibitionistic fashion. They are also impatient, arrogant, and hypersensitive. Interpersonally, they are exploitative and use others to indulge themselves and their desires. Their behavior is socially facile, pleasant, and endearing. However, they are unable to respond to others with true empathy. When stressed, they can be disdainful, exploitative, and generally irresponsible in their behavior.

Their thinking style is one of cognitive expansiveness and exaggeration. They tend to focus on images and themes rather than on facts and issues. They take liberties with the facts, distort them, and even engage in prevarication and self-deception to preserve their own illusions about themselves and the projects in which they are involved. Their cognitive style is also marked by inflexibility. In addition, they have an exaggerated sense of self-importance and establish unrealistic goals of power, wealth, and ability. They justify all of this with their sense of entitlement and exaggerated sense of their own self-importance.

Their feeling or affective style is characterized by an aura of self-confidence and nonchalance, which is present in most situations, except when their narcissistic confidence is shaken. Then they are likely to respond to criticism with rage. Their feelings toward others vacillate between overidealization and devaluation. Finally, their inability to show empathy is reflected in their superficial relationships, with minimal emotional ties or commitments.

The following two case examples illustrate the differences between the narcissistic personality style (Mr. J.) and the narcissistic personality disorder (Mr. C.).

Table 7.1
A Comparison of the Narcissistic Personality Style and Personality Disorder

Personality Style	Personality Disorder
• Although emotionally vulnerable to negative assessments and feelings of others, they can hurdle these with style and grace.	• React to criticism with feelings of rage, stress, or humiliation (even if not expressed).
• Shrewd in dealing with others, utilizing the strengths and advantages of others to achieve their own goals.	• Interpersonally exploitative, taking advantage of others to achieve their own ends.
• Can energetically sell themselves, their ideas, and their projects.	• Grandiose sense of self-importance.
• Tend to be able competitors who love getting to the top and enjoy staying there.	• Believe their problems are unique and understood only by other special people.
• Can visualize themselves as the best or most accomplished in their field.	• Preoccupied by fantasies of unlimited success, power, brilliance, beauty, or ideal love.
• They believe in themselves, their abilities, and their uniqueness, but do not demand special treatment or privileges.	• Have a sense of entitlement and unreasonable expectations of especially favorable treatment.
• Accept accomplishments, praise, and admiration gracefully and with self-possession.	• Require constant attention and admiration.
• Possess a keen awareness of their thoughts and feelings, and have some awareness of those of others.	• Lack empathy; unable to recognize and experience how others feel.
• Expect others to treat them well at all times.	• Preoccupied with feelings of envy.

Case Study: Narcissistic Personality Disorder

Mr. C. is a 41-year-old man who presented for therapy after his wife of six years threatened to leave him and because his employer was pressuring him to resign his position as a sales executive for a condominium project. Apparently, Mrs. C. had told her husband that he loved himself "a hundred times more than you love me." Mr. C. countered this by saying that he needed to buy $600 suits because his job demanded that he look his best at all times, and that he was "tall, dark, handsome, and sexy, all any woman could want in a man." Mr. C. denied that he used scare tactics, exaggerated claims, or other pressure selling techniques with customers. "Sure, I'm a bit aggressive, but you don't get into the 'millionaires' club' by being a wimp." He added that his employer would "go belly up without me," and that he was too important to be dismissed for such petty reasons.

Case Study: Narcissistic Personality Style

Mr. J. is the chairman of his state's Democratic party and caucus. Through-out most of his career, Mr. J. has been incredibly successful and effective. He is extroverted, witty, and charming interpersonally, and astute, vision-ary, and effective in mobilizing support for his party's political agenda. While he was in graduate school, however, a political science professor had criticized a first draft of his master's thesis, evaluating his arguments as weak and his conclusions as only partially substantiated by the research cited. Prior to this, he had held the professor in high esteem, but ques-tioned his competence after the criticism. Nevertheless, he swallowed his pride and reworked the thesis according to the professor's suggestions, and graduated. A short time after graduation, Mr. J. lost his first job as a speech writer for a state senator because the opinions and conclusions cited in his drafts were not sufficiently well documented. He took these lessons to heart and found others to research his speeches when he ran for office. Mr. J. recognized that this was not one of his strengths, and that he could delegate it while focusing on his real strengths, which were envisioning policy and political agendas and galvanizing support for them.

DSM-IV Description and Criteria

According to DSM-IV, the narcissistic personality disorder involves a per-vasive pattern of grandiosity (in fantasy or behavior), a need for admira-tion, and a lack of empathy, beginning by early adulthood and present in a variety of contexts. It is indicated by at least five of the nine criteria listed in Table 7.2.

FORMULATIONS OF NARCISSISTIC PERSONALITY DISORDER

Psychodynamic Formulation

Freud (1914/1976) described the original psychoanalytic formulation of narcissistic personality. For Freud, parental overvaluation or erratic, unre-liable caretaking in early life disrupted the development of object love in

Table 7.2
DSM-IV Criteria for Narcissistic Personality Disorder*

301.81 Narcissistic Personality Disorder

A pervasive pattern of grandiosity (in fantasy or behavior), need for admiration, and lack of empathy, beginning by early adulthood and present in a variety of contexts, as indicated by five (or more) of the following:

(1) has a grandiose sense of self-importance (e.g., exaggerates achievements and talents, expects to be recognized as superior without commensurate achievements)

(2) is preoccupied with fantasies of unlimited success, power, brilliance, beauty, or ideal love

(3) believes that he or she is "special" and unique and can only be understood by, or should associate with, other special or high-status people (or institutions)

(4) requires excessive admiration

(5) has a sense of entitlement, i.e., unreasonable expectations of especially favorable treatment or automatic compliance with his or her expectations

(6) is interpersonally exploitative, i.e., takes advantage of others to achieve his or her own ends

(7) lacks empathy: is unwilling to recognize or identify with the feelings and needs of others

(8) is often envious of others or believes that others are envious of him or her

(9) shows arrogant, haughty behaviors or attitudes

*Reprinted with permission from the *Diagnostic and Statistical Manual of Mental Disorders, Fourth Edition.* Copyright 1994 American Psychiatric Association.

the child. Freud posited that as a result of this fixation or arrest at the narcissistic phase of development, narcissists would be unable to form lasting relationships.

In the past two decades, the formulations of the narcissistic personality by Kohut and Kernberg have become the dominant models. Kohut (1971, 1977) believed that narcissists are developmentally arrested at the stage that requires specific responses from individuals in their environment to maintain cohesive selves; that is, the structures of the grandiose self and the idealized parental image are not integrated. He described the formulation of self-object transferences—both mirroring and idealizing—that recreate the situation with the parents that was not fully successful during childhood. When such responses are not forthcoming (an empathic deficit), the narcissist is prone to fragmentation of the self (narcissistic injury).

Unlike Kohut, who worked with highly functioning professionals in psychoanalysis, Kernberg (1975, 1984) based his conceptualization of narcissistic pathology on his work with both inpatients and outpatients. He views the narcissist's grandiosity and exploitation as evidence of oral rage, which, he believes, results from the emotional deprivation caused by on indifferent and covertly spiteful mother figure. Concurrently, some unique attribute, talent, or role provides the child with a sense of being special, which provides an emotional escape valve in a world of perceived threat or indifference. Thus grandiosity and entitlement shelter a "real self" that is "split off," that is, is outside consciousness. Parenthetically for Kernberg, the real self contains strong but unconscious feelings of envy, deprivation, fear, and rage. Finally, Kernberg (1975) views the defensive structure of the narcissist as remarkably similar to that of the borderline, differentiating the two on the basis of the narcissist's integrated but pathological grandiose self.

Biosocial Formulation

According to Millon and Everly (1985), the narcissistic personality disorder primarily arises from environmental factors, since the role of biogenic factors is unclear. The principal environmental factors are parental indulgence and overvaluation, learned exploitative behavior, and only-child status. Essentially then, children are pampered and given special treatment by the parents, and so learn to believe that the world revolves around them. They become egotistical in their perspectives and narcissistic in their expressions of love and emotion. Not surprisingly, they come to expect special treatment from others outside the home. When this special treatment is not forthcoming, the children experiment with demanding and exploitative tactics, and subsequently develop considerable skill in manipulating others so as to receive the special consideration they believe they deserve. At the same time, they come to believe that most others are inferior, weak, and exploitable. Furthermore, Millon and Everly write that parental overindulgence is particularly likely with only children. Finally, the narcissistic pattern is self-perpetuated through their illusion of their superiority, a lack of self-control manifest in their disdain for persons and situations that do not support their exalted beliefs, deficient social responsibility, and self-reinforcement of the narcissistic pattern itself.

Cognitive-Behavioral Formulation

According to Beck et al. (1990), narcissistic personality disorder stems from a combination of schemas about the self, the world, and the future. The central schema is the superior/special schema, which develops as a result of direct and indirect messages from parents, siblings, and significant others, as well as of experiences that mold beliefs about personal uniqueness and self-importance. The schema of being superior can be shaped by flattery, indulgence, and favoritism. Similarly, the schema of being special can be shaped by experiences of rejection, limitations, exclusion, or deficits. The common denominator for such beliefs about self is that the individual perceives himself or herself as different from others in significant ways. The actual presence of some culturally valued—or devalued—talent or attribute tends to elicit social responses that reinforce the superior/special schema. Feedback that could modify this schema may be lacking or distorted. Being insulated from negative feedback may contribute to the narcissistic vulnerability to criticism and evaluation. Behavior is affected by difficulty in cooperation and reciprocal social intervention and by excesses in self-indulgent, demanding, and aggressive behavior. Problems emerge when this self-schema is overactive and is not balanced by more integrative judgments.

Interpersonal Formulation

For Benjamin (1993), persons with narcissistic personality disorders typically were raised in an environment of selfless, noncontingent love and adoration. Unfortunately, this adoration was not accompanied by genuine self-disclosure. As a result, the narcissistic personality-to-be learned to be unsensitive to others' needs and views. The adoring parent is likely to have been consistently differential and nurturant to the narcissist-in-training. As a result, the adult narcissist holds the arrogant expectation that others will continue to provide these emotional supplies. Along with this nurturance and adoration is the ever-present threat of a fall from grace. As such, the narcissistic individual who is simply "normal" and ordinary creates unbearable disappointment for the parents. Thus the burden of being special or perfect can be overwhelming for the narcissistic individual. Since this individual's self-concept derives from an internalization of unrealistic adoration and nurturance, the substitution of criticism or disappointment for love can be particularly devastating. The narcissistically disordered individual can "dish it out," but is not well equipped "to take it." In short, there is extreme vulnerability to criticism or being ignored, together with a strong wish for love, support, and admiration from others. Noncontingent love from and presumptive control of others are expected, and even demanded. If support is withdrawn or lack of perfection is evident, the self-concept degrades into severe self-criticism. Totally devoid of empathy, these individuals tend to treat others with contempt and rage if entitlement fails.

Integrative Formulation

The following integrative formulation may be helpful in understanding how the narcissistic personality developed and is maintained.

Biologically narcissistic personalities tend to have hyperresponsive temperaments (Millon, 1981). As young children, they were viewed by others as being special in terms of looks, talents, or "promise." Often as young children they had early and exceptional speech development. In addition, they were likely keenly aware of interpersonal cues.

Psychologically, the narcissists' views of themselves, others, the world, and life's purpose can be articulated in terms of the following themes: "I'm special and unique, and I am entitled to extraordinary rights and privileges whether I have earned them or not." Their world view is a variant of the theme: "Life is a banquet table to be sampled at will. People owe me

Table 7.3
Characteristics of Narcissistic Personality Disorder

1. Behavioral appearance	Conceited, boastful, snobbish; self-assured, self-centered, pompous; impatient, arrogant, thin-skinned
2. Interpersonal behavior	Disdainful, exploitative, irresponsible; socially facile but without empathy; uses others to indulge himself or herself
3. Cognitive style	Cognitive expansiveness and exaggeration; focus on images and themes—takes liberties with facts; persistent and inflexible; defense is projective identification
4. Feeling style	Self-confidence; narcissistic rage
5. Parental injunction/ environmental factors	"Grow up and be wonderful, for me."
6. Biological/temperament	Special looks, talents, or "promise"; early and exceptional language development
7. Self view	"I'm special and unique, and I'm entitled to extraordinary rights and privileges whether I've earned them or not."
8. World view	"Life is a banquet table to be sampled at will. People owe me admiration and privilege. Therefore, I'll expect and demand this specialness."
9. Self and system perpetuant	Illusion of specialness (+) disdain for others' views (+) entitlement→ underdeveloped social interest and responsibility→ increased self-absorption and reinforcement of narcissistic style

admiration and privilege." Their goal is: "Therefore, I'll expect and demand this specialness." Common defense mechanisms utilized by the narcissistic personality involve rationalization and projective identification.

Socially, predictable parental patterns and environmental factors can be noted for the narcissistic personality, which is characterized by parental indulgence and overvaluation. The parental injunction likely was: "Grow up and be wonderful—for me." Often they were only children, and, in addition, may have sustained early losses in childhood. From an early age, they learned exploitative and manipulative behavior from their parents. This narcissistic pattern is confirmed, reinforced, and perpetuated by certain individual and systems factors. The illusion of specialness, disdain for others' views, and a sense of entitlement lead to an underdeveloped sense of social interest and responsibility. This, in turn, leads to increased self-absorption and confirmation of narcissistic beliefs (Sperry & Mosak, 1993).

ASSESSMENT OF NARCISSISTIC PERSONALITY DISORDER

Several sources of information are useful in establishing a diagnosis and treatment plan for personality disorders. Observation, collateral information, and psychological testing are important adjuncts to the patient's self-report in the clinical interview. This section briefly describes some characteristic observations that the clinician makes and the nature of the rapport likely to develop in initial encounters with specific personality-disordered individuals. Characteristic response patterns on various objective (i.e., MMPI-2 and MCMI-II) and projective (i.e., Rorschach and TAT) tests are also described.

Interviewing individuals with narcissistic personality disorders is singularly different from interviewing other personality-disordered individuals. Throughout the interview, these individuals give clinicians the impression that the interview has only one purpose: to endorse their self-promoted importance (Othmer & Othmer, 1989). They typically present as self-assured, pretentious, and unwilling to adapt to the basic cultural differences customary to the patient role. They behave as though they are indifferent to the clinician's perspective. As long as the clinician plays the expected role, he or she is idealized as a marvelous clinician. However, confronting their grandiosity early in the treatment process inevitably will lead to rage, and possibly to premature termination. They prefer open-ended questions that permit them to give extended descriptions of their many talents, accomplishments, and future plans. Rapport is established after a considerable period of mirroring and soothing. Typical clinician countertransferences in the initial interviews are boredom, frustration, and anger. To the extent that the clinician can patiently wait through this period of mirroring, the work of confronting and interpreting the narcissists' grandiosity can begin.

This section describes typical themes and patterns noted for the narcissistic personality on the Minnesota Multiphasic Personality Inventory (MMPI-2), the Millon Clinical Multiaxial Inventory (MCMI-II), the Rorschach Psychodiagnostic Test, and the Thematic Apperception Test (TAT). These data have been useful in diagnosing the narcissistic personality disorder, as well as the narcissistic personality style or trait.

On the MMPI-2, a 4-9 (Psychopathic Deviant–Hypomania) profile or an elevation on scale 4 is most likely. Since they develop only superficial relationships, a low score on 0 (Social Introversion) might also be noted. And since they often fit stereotypic sexual roles, scale 5 (Masculinity–Femininity) may be low, particularly for narcissistic men. If they also tend to be suspicious or irritable, an elevation on scale 6 (Paranoia) may be noted (Meyer, 1993).

On the MCMI-II, elevation on scale 5 (Narcissistic) is expected. Scales 4 (Histrionic), 6A (Antisocial), and 6B (Sadistic) could also be elevated. During periods of stress, elevations on P (Paranoid) and DD (Delusional Disorder) may be noted. Since these individuals are averse to admitting psychic distress or personal weakness, elevations on scales A (Anxiety), D (Dysthymia), and S (Schizotypal) are not likely (Choca et al., 1992).

On the Rorschach, these individuals are likely to produce records with a high number of C (Pure Color) and CF (Color Form) responses. They seldom respond directly to shading (Y, YF, or FY), but often make texture (T, TF, or FT) responses (Meyer, 1993). Responses that reflect the ornate, the exotic, or the expensive are characteristics of narcissism (Shafer, 1954).

On the TAT, these individuals tend to avoid the essential features of the cards, and thus their stories may be devoid of meaningful content. Cards that demand a response to potentially anxiety-producing fantasy, such as 13 MF, may yield a superficially avoidant story or one with blatant shocking or lewd content (Bellak, 1993).

TREATMENT APPROACHES AND INTERVENTIONS

Treatment Considerations

Included in the differential diagnosis of the narcissistic personality disorder are these other Axis II personality disorders: histrionic personality disorder, antisocial personality disorder, and paranoid personality disorder. The most common Axis I syndromes associated with the narcissistic personality disorder are acute anxiety reactions, dysthymia, hypochondriasis, and delusional disorders.

In terms of treatment goals, a decision needs to be made as to whether the treatment is to be short term and crisis oriented or long term and focused on personality restructuring. Crisis-oriented psychotherapy usually focuses on alleviation of the symptoms, such as anxiety, depression, or the somatic symptoms associated with the narcissistic injury or wound. The goals of longer-term therapy often involve the restructuring of personality. They include increasing empathy, decreasing rage and cognitive distortions, and increasing the individual's ability to mourn losses. The following sections describe various treatment approaches and individual, group, marital and family, medication, and combined integrative formats.

INDIVIDUAL PSYCHOTHERAPIES

Alone, or in conjunction with group or marital and family therapy, individual psychotherapy is viewed by many as the basic treatment of choice for individuals with narcissistic personality disorder. Because of their empathic deficit and proclivity to devaluing others, psychotherapy with these individuals can be very trying. The fact that they give little, treat others shabbily, and demand much tends to frustrate the natural inclination of therapists to respond empathically. And although the literature is divided over whether to utilize confrontation or mirroring techniques, both approaches must be part of the therapist's armamentarium. Generally speaking, higher functioning narcissistic personalities eventually do well in psychotherapy as their sense of entitlement gives way to emulation. But lower functioning narcissistic personalities have fewer of the necessary personality assets and relational skills for changing, and unless the therapeutic process addresses these deficits, they may leave treatment precipitously to avoid the humiliation of admitting how ill equipped they are to achieve realistic treatment goals. Psychodynamic, cognitive-behavioral, and interpersonal approaches are briefly described.

Psychodynamic Psychotherapy Approach

This section briefly outlines the various psychodynamic approaches: psychoanalysis, psychoanalytic psychotherapy, supportive psychotherapy, and brief psychoanalytic psychotherapy.

Psychoanalysis

Although Freud (1914/1976) was not optimistic about the treatability of the narcissistic personality, Kernberg (1984) and Kohut (1971) believe that higher functioning patients with narcissistic personality disorders are particularly suited for psychoanalysis. Kernberg views the core of the disorder as involving anger, envy, and distorted self-sufficiency, and so emphasizes an active interpretation and confrontation of the individual's defenses.

Kohut, on the other hand, views the core of the disorder as stunted development of the grandiose self. He believes that through the establishment of a self-object transference, both mirroring and idealizing, missing elements of the self-structure can be added. When a correct empathic interpretation is made, the individual reintegrates by way of the reestablishment of the self-object transference—cohesion—and the disappearance of fragmentation. In short then, Kernberg's goal of psychoanalysis is to effect a significant personality change so that envy and rage no longer overwhelm the individual and lead to a protective need to withdraw to a self-sufficient position. For Kohut, the goal is to heal the individual's incomplete self-structure and to increase self-esteem through transmuting internalization, that is, the taking in of missing functions from the self-object analysis. The process of psychoanalysis for both Kohut and Kernberg is expected to take several years because significant personality change is the goal.

Psychoanalytic Psychotherapy

In what he calls expressive psychotherapy, Kernberg (1984) describes a modified psychoanalytic treatment as an alternative to psychoanalysis and supportive psychotherapy. In expressive psychotherapy, the therapeutic effort focuses on the negative transference in which early manifestations of anger toward the therapist are explored and interpreted. Also included are the defenses of splitting, projection, and projective identification. Masterson (1981) and Rinsley (1982) further emphasize the value of this approach in the development of a therapeutic alliance. Masterson also emphasizes the importance of exploring the individual's exquisite sensitivity to the therapist's empathic failures and the importance of exploring this vulnerability therapeutically. Although Kohut did not describe a psychotherapeutic treatment of the narcissistic personality disorder, Goldberg (1973) and Chessick (1985) have shown that self-object transferences do become established in psychotherapy and can be interpreted in light of Kohut's approach. Goldberg (1989) describes the use of the mirroring, idealizing, and twinship transference in a self psychology approach with the narcissistic patient.

Psychoanalytically oriented psychotherapy of narcissistically disordered individuals typically involves one to three sessions a week for two or more years. Kantor (1992) offers a number of proactive suggestions for use in the course of psychotherapy. Among them is the use of predictive interpretation. He points out how painful therapy will be as the patient feels forced to abandon his or her entitlement and grandiosity. With such forewarning, the person is less likely to leave therapy precipitously.

Supportive Psychotherapy

According to Kernberg (1984), supportive psychotherapy emphasizes avoiding working with the negative transference, and instead focusing on supporting the individual in developing expanding ego functions, skills, and capacities. According to Kernberg, rapid symptomatic improvement is more likely in supportive psychotherapy than in more expressive approaches. The reader is referred to Kernberg's (1984) chapter on "Supportive Psychotherapy" for an extended discussion of treatment goals and techniques. Kantor (1992) recommends palliation as the goal of supportive psychotherapy, wherein the disordered narcissistic personality is maintained while reducing or eliminating its destructive sequelae. He recommends a number of palliative strategies, such as teaching the individual to become a better narcissist. For instance, Kantor shows how excessive self-adoration actually interferes with the ability to receive more realistic, wanted, and needed adoration from others.

Brief Psychoanalytically Oriented Psychotherapy
Not surprisingly, the least explored treatment modalities of the psychodynamic therapies of the narcissistic personality disorder are the shorter-term and brief approaches. Until recently, a self-deficit disorder such as the narcissistic personality was considered unamenable to any but long-term treatment. However, as economic realities collide with ideology, this view may be changing somewhat. Kernberg (1984) describes a short-term crisis intervention for the narcissistic personality disorder that can be used until the individual is ready and motivated for long-term treatment. Lazarus (1982) and Binder (1979) report utilizing a brief approach for increasing the individual's self-esteem and self-cohesion, again as preparation for longer-term treatment. Klein (1989b) describes a short-term treatment that is not a preparation for longer-term therapy. Admittedly, the goals are not ego repair, but are more limited. They include learning, or an increased awareness and anticipation of personal vulnerability to injury, shame, and disappointment; containment, or an increased ability to modulate affects, especially narcissistic rage; and adaptation, that is, seriously taking into account those aspects of reality previously ignored and their destructive consequences. Interpretation of narcissistic vulnerability and clarification of the need for containment of defensive devaluation and withdrawal are the cornerstones of this approach. Klein, a colleague of Masterson, describes two selection criteria: (1) an acute interruption of narcissistic "supply lives" (i.e., interpersonal rejection or disappointment), resulting in narcissistic injury amenable to a substitute "supply line" (i.e., the therapist's mirroring); and (2) when the narcissistic injury makes conscious a persistent vulnerability (often experienced as depression or somatic preoccupation) and these individuals are motivated to learn more adaptive ways of managing their environment. Klein specifically excludes from his brief approach those who present or are referred with chronic, nonspecific, vague, or ego-syntonic symptoms. He describes a course of time-limited treatment (i.e., six months) with a young man that effected symptom relief and a circumscribed im-

provement in functioning. Oldham (1988) presents a 24-session treatment strategy that he describes as a dynamically informed directive approach with limited, focused treatment goals. Marmar and Freeman (1988) also describe a brief dynamic approach.

Cognitive-Behavioral Approach

Beck et al. (1990) provide an in-depth discussion of the cognitive therapy approach to patients with narcissistic personality disorders. Early in the course of therapy with these individuals, three treatment objectives must be met: developing a collaborative working relationship, socializing the individuals to the cognitive theory and model of treatment, and agreeing on treatment goals. Forming a collaborative relationship is challenging in that narcissists are deeply invested in being special and superior, and usually have a limited capacity for working collaboratively. Establishing and maintaining firm treatment guidelines and limits in a neutral, matter-of-fact tone is necessary. It should be pointed out that sticking to an agreed-upon agenda allows the therapist to address the narcissistic individual's important concerns more effectively. Similarly, the therapist can approach, other counterproductive behaviors in therapy by appealing to the person's self-interest.

Because disclosing shortcomings and weaknesses is alien to the narcissist's style, behavioral interventions are usually easier to implement earlier in treatment since they require less self-disclosure than do most cognitive techniques. The rhythm of treatment with narcissistic individuals alternates focus among increasing responsibility for behavior; decreasing cognitive distortions and dysfunctional affects, such as rage reactions; and, developing healthier attitudes and beliefs. The challenge with these individuals is to tailor treatment to the three components of grandiosity, hypersensitivity to criticism, and empathic deficits. Cognitive techniques are useful in revising their distorted self-views, particularly with dichotomous, black–white thinking. Furthermore, magical restructuring methods wherein a realistic and pleasurable fantasy replaces a grandiose one are also useful. Systematic desensitization and role reversal can be used to address hypersensitivity. Working with empathy deficits is a major focus of treatment and involves several techniques. After bringing these deficits to the attention of the individual, emotional schemas related to the feelings and reactions of others are activated, usually through role plays, including role reversal. Then alternative ways of relating to others can be discussed, and new statements of belief, such as "others' feelings count too," are formulated. The use of significant others in therapy—as in couples sessions—has been found of use in developing and practicing empathy and in reinforcing changes, as well as in helping the significant other to cope more effectively with the narcissistic individual. In summary, cognitive therapy with persons with narcissistic personality disorders can be most challenging; nevertheless, it can help them to make significant changes. Beck indicates that the best predictors of success are the degree of narcissism and the therapist's ability to withstand the individual's demands for approval and special treatment. To the extent that a collaborative working relationship is established, limits are set and maintained regarding the control of therapy and special treatment, and schemas of regarding grandiosity, hypersensitivity, and empathy are changed and associated behaviors and affects modulated, positive treatment outcomes are likely.

Interpersonal Approach

For Benjamin (1993), psychotherapeutic interventions with persons with narcissistic personality disorders can be planned and evaluated in terms of whether they enhance collaboration, facilitate learning about maladaptive patterns and their roots, block these patterns, enhance the will to change, and effectively encourage new patterns.

Facilitating collaboration with narcissistic individuals is rooted in accurate, consistent empathy. Consistent empathy provides the affirmation and soothing needed to learn self-regulation. Through the experience of being accurately mirrored, the person is able to internalize this empathic affirmation of self. Another important aspect of collaboration involves the individual's learning to tolerate his or her faults. This is facilitated through modeling as the therapist acknowledges mistakes or errors, such as an occasional minor lapse in understanding the individual. In therapy, narcissistic individuals must learn to recognize and block the patterns of entitlement, grandiosity, and envy of others' success. Gentle confrontations embedded in strong support are utilized for this purpose. To accomplish this successfully, the therapist must master the delicate art of pushing the edge of awareness without destroying the therapeutic relationship. Couples therapy can be useful in the recognition and blocking of maladaptive patterns.

Once these individuals understand their maladaptive patterns and choose to relinquish the quest for unattainable or maladaptive goals, new learning is relatively easy. According to Benjamin, the basic focus of interpersonal learning is empathy. Empathy can be effectively taught in couples therapy. Role playing and other empathy training approaches can be particularly useful. Benjamin contends that when utilizing role playing, it is important that a collaborative and benign use of the individual's exact words and inflections be employed, as inexact mirroring can elicit rage and withdrawal.

GROUP THERAPY

There is a growing literature on the treatment of people with narcissistic personality disorders in group therapy formats. Many of the recent reports are based on object-relations or self- psychology approaches (Leszcz, 1989). Outcome research demonstrates that group therapy is as effective as any other therapy in treating the narcissistic personality disorder (Alonso, 1992). A number of factors contribute to the effectiveness of groups with this personality disorder. First, peer rather than therapist feedback is likely to be more acceptable to the individual. Second, transferences are likely to be less intense than in individual therapy. Working through intense affects is possible because of the individual's positive attachments within the group and because of peer group scrutiny of the person's disavowed affects. Third, group membership provides the narcissistic individual with three unique requirements: mirroring of needs, objects for idealization, and opportunities for peer relationships (Grotjahn, 1984). Finally, the group provides individuals with opportunities to increase their capacity to empathize with others, as well as to enhance self-esteem and self-cohesion.

Most of the recent reports suggest that groups consisting exclusively of narcissistic individuals can have successful therapeutic outcomes. Alonso (1992) notes that while narcissistic pathology undermines the usual forces that lead to group cohesion, a properly run group can function as a container for splitting and oscillation of self-love and hate. She also notes that a high dropout rate is common in groups for those with narcissistic personality disorders with as many as 50 percent dropping out of ongoing—rather than time-limited—groups. Alonso recommends intermittent individual therapy focused on helping people remain in the group. Horowitz (1977) describes the indications for and contraindications to group treatment of narcissistic individuals. He notes four indications: demandingness, egocentrism, social isolation and withdrawal, and socially deviant behavior. Even though these traits may be taxing for both the therapist and group members, Horowitz believes individuals with such traits are quite amenable to group treatment. Finally, Stone and Whiteman (1980) note that attention to the unique needs of the individual might warrant a deemphasis on interpretations geared to the entire group and a focus on an individual member's needs or capacities that are different from those of the group.

MARITAL/FAMILY THERAPY

The early family-therapy literature emphasized the treatment of adolescents in families with severe narcissistic pathology (Shapiro, 1982; Berkowitz, Shapiro, Sinner, et al., 1974). Typically, such families identify the adolescent as the patient and project onto him or her their own deval-ued views of themselves. Not surprisingly, when the adolescent attempts to separate and individualize, the parent's rage and projections intensify. In a family therapy format, the therapist functions to contain displaced, projected, and acted-out impulses and affects. Furthermore, the therapist must acknowledge, work through, and redirect these responses, and so provide the family with an opportunity to restore previously severed com-munication and mutual support during this critical phase of adolescent development.

More recent applications of family therapy to the narcissistic personal-ity disorder treat entire family systems or one or both parents/spouses. Jones (1987) advocates a family systems approach to the narcissistic family. He suggests several strategies, in particular, determining the dilemma the family faces regarding change by analyzing the metaphorical themes that paradoxically bind the family to resist change. Subsequently, the therapist must join—rather than challenge or confront—the family's resistance. Such an empathic relationship is useful in understanding how resistance can be lowered. Usually, family sessions are scheduled weekly for 90 minutes with all family members present. Such family treatment has been described as lasting up to or more than a year.

Considerably more has been published about marital therapy with the narcissistic spouse or couple. Berkowitz (1985) has described a couples therapy protocol based on Kohut's view of narcissistic vulnerability, self-object needs, and projective identification. The couple is seen conjointly in weekly sessions—usually 75 to 90 minutes—with the goal of "owning" projections and internalizing needed self-object functions. Lachkar (1986, 1992) describes a common spousal bond: the narcissist dominated by mir-roring needs and the others by fears of abandonment. She describes a psy-choanalytic treatment approach, combining both object relations theory and self psychology, in which the therapist functions as a self-object so that the exhibitionistic/bonding expectations can be channeled into seeking more realistic goals. Therapy is envisioned as involving three developmental phases: fusion, separation, and interaction. It should be noted that Lachkar views conjoint marital therapy as a precursor to individual psychotherapy or psychoanalysis of one or both spouses. Furthermore, she adds that in conjoint work the therapeutic alliance must be joined by the spouse who is predominately narcissistic because of his or her tendency to flee, become isolated, and withdraw from therapy.

Solomon (1989) discusses marital therapy wherein one or both spouses meet the criteria for the narcissistic personality disorder. Elucidating a self-psychology perspective of narcissism in marriage, she describes a conjoint treatment protocol where marital therapy sessions function as a "holding environment." Furthermore, she believes that distorted conscious and unconscious communication is central to marital conflict and its resolution. Finally, she describes the therapist's empathic self as the basic tool of treatment. Masterson and Orcutt (1989) present a conjoint approach to working with the narcissistic couple.

Relationship enhancement (RE) therapy has been adapted to couples therapy with narcissistic spouses (Snyder, 1994). This therapy is a unique blending of object relationship theory, social learning theory, interpersonal theory, and system theory that provides a psychoeducational format for incorporating skill training in either an individual psychotherapy or conjoint couples therapy.

Relationship enhancement couples therapy focuses on the learning and application of four interpersonal skills: empathy; effective expression; discussion, or mode switching between empathic and expressor roles; and problem solving/conflict resolution. The therapist explains, demonstrates, and coaches each skill in the conjoint session, and the spouse then practices these skills during and between sessions with progressively difficult issues. Not surprisingly, the empathic skills and the subjective aspect of the expressor skill are notably deficient for the narcissistically vulnerable couple. Furthermore, the therapist provides a holding environment in which narcissistic vulnerability is minimally acted out and instead is experienced and addressed productively. As a result, both spouses learn to express their feelings with less risk of shaming the other and are more able to empathize with the feelings of the other spouse that previously evoked defensive reactions. Snyder (1994) provides a detailed case example of this promising approach.

MEDICATION

At present, there is only a small literature defining the use of psychopharmacological agents for the treatment of narcissistic personality disorder. Klein's (1975) discussion of the use of monoamine oxidase inhibitors in hysteroid dysphoria might have relevance to narcissistic personality disorder because both disorders share an exquisite sensitivity to criticism. More recently, Siever (1993) reported preliminary data showing that selective serotonergic reuptake inhibitors such as fluoxetine and sertroline have been effective in reducing the target symptom of interpersonal sensitivity and reactivity.

Abramson (1983) has described the successful use of lorazepam as an adjunct to individual psychotherapy for the treatment of narcissistic rage in three individuals judged as meeting the criteria for narcissistic personality disorder. Reich (1988) reported research showing a strong negative association among a cohort of individuals with panic disorder and narcissistic personality disorder who were treated with benzodiazepines.

Other medications may be utilized successfully with narcissistic individuals with specific target symptoms. An episode of major depression would certainly be a reasonable indication for a trycyclic or newer class of antidepressant, particularly if insomnia is also present.

COMBINED/INTEGRATIVE TREATMENT APPROACHES

As noted in the opening chapter of this book, there is seldom a single treatment of choice, be it a specific method (i.e., mirroring) or a general approach (i.e., psychoanalysis), that can ensure positive treatment outcomes with personality-disordered individuals. Instead, depending on the individual's overall level of functioning, temperamental patterns, defensive style, and skill deficits, a focused, specific, and sequentially coordinated tailored treatment protocol is usually necessary to accomplish treatment goals and objectives in a timely manner.

Several treatment approaches and interventions applicable to narcissistic personality disorder have now been described by orientation (i.e., psychodynamic, cognitive behavioral/psychoeducational, interpersonal) or format (i.e., individual, group, marital/family, or medication). This final section offers another treatment perspective: an integrative and combined approach. Again, as described in the opening chapter, the most highly functioning individuals who meet either DSM-IV or dynamic criteria for a personality disorder are more likely to have fewer troubling temperamental patterns, skill deficits, and defensive styles than the lower functioning individual. And, to repeat the basic premise of this book, the higher the functioning and the fewer skill deficits the personality-disordered individual has, the more likely it is that a single approach will be effective. Conversely, the lower the functioning and the more skill deficits and under- or overmodulated temperament patterns the personality-disordered individual exhibits, the more an integrative, tailored, and combined sequential approach is necessary.

The following are specific treatment strategies and methods aimed at the treatment targets of cognitive style and content, behavioral style, emotional style, and relational style that I have found useful in my clinical and consulting practice. These strategies are based on the following composite model of the narcissistic personality.

This basic stress–diathesis model has narcissistic vulnerability and expectations as the diathesis and the underempathic behavior of others as the stressor. Generally speaking, the psychodynamic approaches have largely emphasized the dimensions of narcissistic vulnerability and narcissistic frustration, focusing particularly on the interpretation of vulnerability regarding grandiosity and entitlement and soothing and mirroring frustrations to reduce narcissistic rage. Largely, the cognitive therapy approaches have focused on modifying narcissistic vulnerability (self and world view), narcissistic expectation, and cognitive distortions. The behavioral and psychoeducational approaches have espoused skill training at several levels, including empathy training (as in relationship enhancement therapy). Finally, the interpersonal approaches emphasize empathy training and appropriate responding to the unempathic behavior of others. Thus no single approach formally affects every level of the model.

I have found it valuable continually to emphasize the dimensions of narcissistic vulnerability throughout treatment, with considerable attention given to the four temperamental styles: cognitive, emotional, relational, and behavioral. For the cognitive style in which the narcissistic individual tends to distort cognitively and to utilize the defenses of splitting and projective identification, cognitive restructuring and cognitive awareness training (Beck et al., 1990) are useful. With regard to emotional style where narcissistic rage is prominent, anger-control training (Turkat, 1990) is indicated. Since empathic deficits greatly affect relational style, empathy training and increasing intimacy-promoting behavior (Snyder, 1994) are indicated. And because narcissistic individuals tend to be impatient and may have difficulty taking responsibility, problem solving, and behavior contracting (Beck et al., 1990) have been found useful. Efforts to effect change in schemas, especially self view and world view, with psychodynamic interpretation and both cognitive restructuring methods are usually necessary. I have found that a successful course of therapy may encompass up to 100 or more sessions. When individual psychotherapy can be combined with group therapy or couples therapy, I have noted that treatment can be greatly facilitated, needing only 30 or so sessions. I am much less optimistic about long-term treatment for the lower functioning narcissist, unless group or couples therapy is mandatory. See Figure 7.2.

Medication seems to be particularly useful when exquisite sensitivity to criticism or impulsivity and anger control are problematic. I have found fluoxetine particularly valuable in these instances.

Figure 7.1
Composite Model of the Narcissistic Personality Disorder

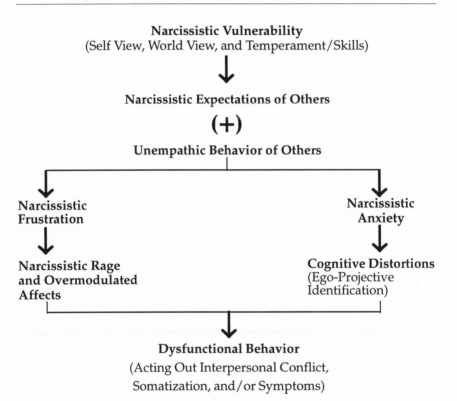

Narcissistic Vulnerability
(Self View, World View, and Temperament/Skills)

↓

Narcissistic Expectations of Others

(+)

Unempathic Behavior of Others

Narcissistic
Frustration

Narcissistic
Anxiety

Narcissistic Rage
and Overmodulated
Affects

Cognitive Distortions
(Ego-Projective
Identification)

Dysfunctional Behavior
(Acting Out Interpersonal Conflict,
Somatization, and/or Symptoms)

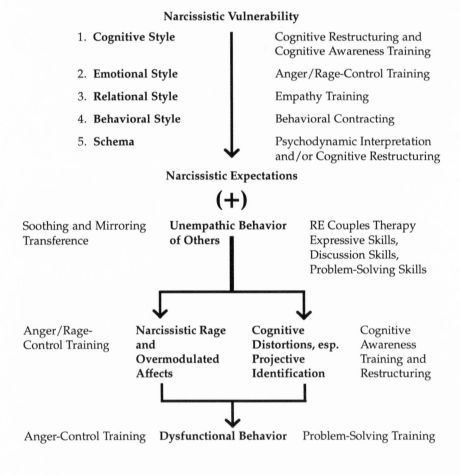

Figure 7.2
Targeted Treatment Interventions for Narcissistic Personality Disorder

Narcissistic Vulnerability

1. **Cognitive Style**   Cognitive Restructuring and
                                 Cognitive Awareness Training

2. **Emotional Style**   Anger/Rage-Control Training

3. **Relational Style**   Empathy Training

4. **Behavioral Style**   Behavioral Contracting

5. **Schema**   Psychodynamic Interpretation
                                 and/or Cognitive Restructuring

Narcissistic Expectations

(+)

Soothing and Mirroring   **Unempathic Behavior**   RE Couples Therapy
Transference   **of Others**   Expressive Skills,
                                                         Discussion Skills,
                                                         Problem-Solving Skills

Anger/Rage-   **Narcissistic Rage**   **Cognitive**   Cognitive
Control Training   **and**   **Distortions, esp.** Awareness
                  Overmodulated   **Projective**   Training and
                  Affects   **Identification**   Restructuring

Anger-Control Training   **Dysfunctional Behavior**   Problem-Solving Training

134

CHAPTER 8

Obsessive-Compulsive Personality Disorder

The obsessive-compulsive personality disorder is distinguished from the obsessive-compulsive disorder in the DSM-III, DSM-III-R, and DSM-IV (Pfohl & Blum, 1991). Whereas individuals with obsessive-compulsive disorder are plagued with recurring unpleasant thoughts and are driven to perform ritualized behaviors that are ego dystonic, those with obsessive-compulsive personality disorder exhibit traits that are adaptive and seldom distressing, and are ego syntonic. Despite these diagnostic differences, some clinicians, particularly psychodynamically oriented ones, note significant similarities between the two. Nemiah (1980) observes that many individuals presenting for psychotherapy with obsessive-compulsive neurotic symptoms also have an underlying obsessive-compulsive character structure, whereas Munich (1986) notes that obsessive-compulsive symptoms are often transitory phenomena during the psychoanalytic treatment of individuals with diagnosed obsessive-compulsive personality disorder. Nevertheless, a distinction is made by DSM-III between Axis I and Axis II obsessive-compulsive presentations, and treatment strategies for the two appear to differ significantly.

135

The estimate is that about 1 percent of the general population would meet the criteria for this disorder. This compares with between 3 and 10 percent of patients in clinical settings.

This chapter describes the characterizing features of the obsessive-compulsive personality disorder and its related personality style. It also describes five clinical formulations of the disorder, psychological assessment indicators, and a variety of treatment approaches, modalities, and intervention strategies.

CHARACTERISTICS OF THE OBSESSIVE-COMPULSIVE PERSONALITY STYLE AND DISORDER

The obsessive-compulsive personality can be thought of as spanning a continuum from healthy to pathological, with the obsessive personality style at the healthy end and the obsessive-compulsive personality disorder at the pathological end. Table 8.1 compares and contrasts differences between the obsessive-compulsive style and disorder.

The obsessive-compulsive personality disorder can be recognized by the following behavioral and interpersonal, cognitive, and emotional styles. Behaviorally, this disorder is characterized by perfectionism. People with the disorder are likely to be workaholics. In addition to being dependable, they tend to be stubborn and possessive. They, like passive-aggressive–disordered individuals, can be indecisive and procrastinating. Interpersonally, they are exquisitely conscious of social rank and status, and modify their behavior accordingly. That is, they tend to be deferential and obsequious to superiors, and haughty and autocratic to subordinates and peers. They can be doggedly insistent that others do things their way, without appreciating or being aware of how the others react to their insistence. At their best, they are polite and loyal to the organizations and ideals they espouse.

Their thinking style can be characterized as constricted and rule based. They have difficulty establishing priorities and perspective. As "detail" people, they often lose sight of the larger project. In other words, they "cannot see the forest for the trees." Because of their indecisiveness and doubts, decision making is difficult. Their mental inflexibility is matched by their nonsuggestible and unimaginative style, suggesting that they have a restricted fantasy life. Like those with passive-aggressive disorders, obsessive-compulsive individuals have conflicts between assertiveness and defiance and between pleasing and obedience, but for different reasons.

Their affective or emotional style is characterized as grim and cheerless. They have difficulty with expressing intimate feelings such as warmth and tenderness, tending to avoid the "softer" feelings, although they may ex-

Table 8.1
A Comparison of the Obsessive-Compulsive Personality Style and Disorder

Personality Style	*Personality Disorder*
• Desire to complete tasks and projects without flaws or errors.	• Perfectionism that interferes with task completion.
• Take pride in doing all jobs or tasks well, including the smallest details.	• Preoccupation with details, rules, lists, order, organization, or schedules to the extent that the major point of the activity is lost.
• Tend to want things to be done "just right" and in a specific manner, but have some tolerance for things being done another way.	• Unreasonable insistence that others submit exactly to their way of doing things, or unreasonable reluctance to allow others to do things because of the conviction that they will not do them correctly.
• Dedicated to work and working hard; capable of intense, single-minded effort.	• Excessive devotion to work and productivity to the exclusion of leisure activities and friendships (not accounted for by obvious economic necessity).
• Carefully consider alternatives and their consequences in making decisions.	• Indecisive: decision making either avoided, postponed, or protracted (but not due to excessive need for advice or reassurance from others).
• Tend to have strong moral principles and strongly desire to do the right thing.	• Overconscientious, scrupulous, and inflexible about matters of morality, ethics, or values.
• No-nonsense individuals who do their work without much emotional expenditure.	• Restructured expression of affection.
• Generally, are careful, thrifty, and cautious, but are able to share from their abundance.	• Lack of generosity in giving time, money, or gifts when no personal gain is likely to result.
• Tend to save and collect objects and are reluctant to discard objects that have, formerly had, or may have value for them.	• Unable to discard worn-out or worthless objects even when they have no sentimental value.

hibit anger, frustration, and irritability quite freely. This grim, feeling-avoidant demeanor shows itself in stilted, stiff relationship behaviors.

The following case examples further illustrate the differences between the obsessive-compulsive personality disorder (Mr. Z.) and the obsessive-compulsive personality style (Mr. C.).

Case Study: Obsessive-Compulsive Personality Disorder

Mr. Z. is a 39-year-old business executive who wanted to begin a course of psychotherapy because he felt his "whole world was closing in." He gave a history of long-standing feelings of dissatisfaction with his marriage, which had worsened in the past two years. He described his wife's increasing demands for time and affection, which he believed was a weakness on her part. His professional life also had become conflicted when his partner of 10 years wanted to expand their accounting firm to another city. Mr. Z. said he believed that this proposal was fraught with danger and he had come to the point of selling his share of the business to his partner. He knew he had to make some decisions about his marriage and his business, but was unable to do so. He said he hoped that therapy would help with these decisions. He presented as neatly dressed in a conservative three-piece blue suit. His posture was rigid, and he spoke in a formal and controlled tone with constricted affect. His thinking was characterized by preoccupation with details and was somewhat circumstantial.

Case Study: Obsessive-Compulsive Personality Style

Mr. C. is a 41-year-old assistant vice president of personnel for a public utility. He rose through the ranks because of his loyalty and accomplishments above and beyond the call of duty. Because of thoroughness and attention to detail, he has saved his corporation nearly $3 million in the past two years on insurance and health benefits for the utility's employees. Most evenings, Mr. C. takes a briefcase full of work home with him. Although he does not mind this intrusion into his family life, his wife of 18 years told him that she did. Accordingly, they reached an agreement that Mr. C. would spend at least two hours with her and their three children before turning to his briefcase.

DSM-IV Description and Criteria

Unlike the Axis I obsessive-compulsive disorder, ritualistic compulsions and obsessions do not characterize the obsessive-compulsive personality disorder. DSM-IV offers the description and criteria shown in Table 8.2

Table 8.2
DSM-IV Description and Criteria for
Obsessive-Compulsive Personality Disorder*

301.4 Obsessive-Compulsive Personality Disorder

A pervasive pattern of preoccupation with orderliness, perfectionism, and mental and interpersonal control, at the expense of flexibility, openness, and efficiency, beginning by early adulthood and present in a variety of contexts, as indicated by four (or more) of the following:

(1) is preoccupied with details, rules, lists, order, organization, or schedules to the extent that the major point of the activity is lost

(2) shows perfectionism that interferes with task completion (e.g., is unable to complete a project because his or her own overly strict standards are not met)

(3) is excessively devoted to work and productivity to the exclusion of leisure activities and friendships (not accounted for by obvious economic necessity)

(4) is overconscientious, scrupulous, and inflexible about matters of morality, ethics, or values (not accounted for by cultural or religious identification)

(5) is unable to discard worn-out or worthless objects even when they have no sentimental value

(6) is reluctant to delegate tasks or to work with others unless they submit to exactly his or her way of doing things

(7) adopts a miserly spending style toward both self and others; money is viewed as something to be hoarded for future catastrophes

(8) shows rigidity and stubbornness

*Reprinted with permission from the *Diagnostic and Statistical Manual of Mental Disorders, Fourth Edition.* Copyright 1994 American Psychiatric Association.

FORMULATIONS OF THE OBSESSIVE-COMPULSIVE PERSONALITY DISORDER

Psychodynamic Formulation

Early psychoanalytic writers formulated the obsessive-compulsive personality as a regression from the oedipal phase to the anal phase of development. Because of a punitive superego, these obsessive-compulsive persons employed intellectualization, isolation of affect, undoing, development, and reaction formation as defenses. Presumably, they experienced difficulty expressing aggression as a result of power struggles with maternal figures over toilet training.

Contemporary writers, however, formulate this pattern as much broader than anal fixation. They contend that as children these individuals were not sufficiently valued or loved by their caretakers, and subsequently developed overwhelming doubt. Salzman (1980) believes that the obsessive pattern is basically a device for preventing any thought or feeling that might produce shame, a loss of pride or status, or a feeling of deficiency or weakness, regardless or whether the feelings are hostile, sexual, or otherwise. He views obsessive compulsivity as a neurotic strategy that protects these individuals from exposing any thoughts or feelings that could endanger their physical or psychological existence. This overriding need to control their inner and outer worlds requires that they lead overly structured and manageable lives. They tend to maintain doubts, are willing to make commitments, and strive for perfection. Thus it is necessary for them to know everything in order to predict the future and prepare for every exigency. To maintain the fiction of perfection, they must never make an error or admit any deficiency. Furthermore, their tendency to procrastinate is related to their tendency to doubt as a means of guaranteeing their omniscience when life forces a decision or choice. As such, they are deeply ambivalent, which allows them to maintain security, but at the price of productivity and positive feelings and attitudes.

These individuals find both anger and dependency consciously unacceptable and so defend against these feelings with such defenses as reaction formation and isolation of affect, as well as differential and obsequious behaviors. Intimacy poses major concerns for these people, who fear being overwhelmed by powerful wishes to be taken care of, while also experiencing the frustration of those wishes along with the fear of being out of control. In addition, they harbor the secret conviction that if they could become perfect, they would finally receive the parental approval and esteem they missed in early life. Finally, psychodynamic writers have noted the unique cognitive style of obsessive-compulsive individuals (Shapiro, 1965; Horowitz, 1988; Horowitz, Marmar, Krupnick, et al., 1984), which is characterized by inner drive, careful attention to detail, lack of spontaneity, and ruminative thinking.

Biosocial Formulation

There is no research evidence as yet that biological predisposing factors underlie this disorder (Millon & Everly, 1985). Nonetheless, clinical observations suggest that many obsessive-compulsive individuals display an anhedonic temperament and tend to be first born in their sibships. Certain environmental factors may be etiologic: parental overcontrol, learned compulsive behavior, and responsibility training. Rather than being overprotective, parents of obsessive-compulsive individuals overcontrol in an attempt to prevent their children from causing trouble for themselves or others, and they are punitive when the child misbehaves or fails to meet expectations. These children learn compulsive behavior directly and indirectly within the family matrix. They learn to avoid punishment by accepting and meeting the demands and expectations of perfectionistic and punitive parents. Furthermore, they learn compulsivity by imitating the compulsive behaviors modeled by one or both parents. As a result, they do not develop the ability to generate options and explore alternatives, and thus fail to function autonomously. Obsessive-compulsive individuals are regularly exposed to conditions that teach them to overvalue a sense of responsibility to others. They are taught to feel guilt when these responsibilities are not met, and shame when they act impulsively or even playfully. They learn to be polite, pleasing, and loyal to superiors. These influences typically yield hard-driving, perfectionistic, and seemingly polite and pleasing individuals who lead rather restricted, tentative, colorless lives.

This obsessive-compulsive pattern is self-perpetuated through an interaction of cognitive and behavioral rigidity; a strict adherence to roles, regulations, and social convention; and a tendency to be highly self-critical. Although their cognitive rigidity does reduce the anxiety associated with flexibility and ambivalence, they tend to lead overstructured, one-sided lives. Self-criticism serves to keep them in line, whereas their striving for perfection reduces opportunities for risk taking and adventure.

Cognitive-Behavioral Formulations

Guidano and Liotti (1983) provide a cognitive formulation of this personality pattern based on three maladaptive schemas: perfectionism, the need for certainty, and the belief that there is an absolute, correct solution for every human problem. Guidano and Liotti note that these individuals received mixed, contradictory messages from at least one parent.

Beck et al. (1990) identify some schemas held by obsessive-compulsive individuals. Perfection: "To be worthwhile, I must avoid making mistakes, because to make a mistake is to fail, which would be intolerable," and "If the perfect course of action is unclear, it is better to do nothing." Control: "I must be perfectly in control of myself and my environment, because loss of control is intolerable and dangerous," "Without my rules and rituals, I'll collapse into an inert pile," and "Magical rituals or obsessive ruminations prevent the occurrence of catastrophes."

Beck et al. also describe typical automatic thoughts of obsessive-compulsive individuals: "I need to get this assignment done perfectly," "I have to do this project myself or it won't be done right," "That person misbehaved and should be punished," and "I should keep these old reports because I might need them some day." In addition to these schemas and automatic thoughts, those with this personality pattern often utilize the cognitive distortions of dichotomous thinking and magnification or catastrophizing.

Turkat (1990) and Turkat and Maisto (1985) suggest a behavioral formulation of this pattern. These individuals are noted to have been reared in families that emphasized productivity and rule following at the expense of emotional expression and interpersonal relationships. Accordingly, they did not acquire adequate levels of empathy skills or skills in interacting with others on an emotional basis.

Interpersonal Formulation

According to Benjamin (1993), persons diagnosed with an obsessive-compulsive personality disorder were likely to have been raised in an atmosphere of unreasonable and relentless coercion to perform correctly and to follow rules regardless of personal cost. As a consequence, obsessive-compulsive individuals have an unbalanced devotion to perfection of self and others. Their parents typically held extremely high expectations for self-control and perfection, and not only punished the children for not being perfect, but gave them little or no reward for success. For the adult, this subsequently resulted in a focus on mistakes and self-criticism. Furthermore, as children, they experienced little warmth in their homes. Laughter, hugging, holding, and other signs of affection were seldom, if ever, modeled. Expressions of feelings were considered dangerous. The adult consequence of this lack of warmth and demand for perfection is social correctness, albeit inaccessibility of feelings. Finally, there is a fear of making mistakes and a penchant for rule following. A quest for order underlies blame and inconsiderate control of others alternating with blind obedience to authority. This stance is supported by excessive self-discipline, restraint of excessive feelings, self-criticism, and a neglect of the self.

Integrative Formulation

The following integrative formulation may be helpful in understanding how the obsessive-compulsive personality disorder is likely to develop and be maintained.

Biologically, these individuals are likely to have exhibited an anhedonic temperament as infants (Millon, 1981). Firstborn children have greater propensity for developing a compulsive style than do their siblings (Toman, 1961).

Psychologically, such persons view themselves, others, the world, and life's purpose in terms of the following themes. They tend to view themselves with some variant of the theme: "I'm responsible if something goes wrong, so I have to be reliable, competent, and righteous." Their world view is some variant of the theme: "Life is unpredictable and expects too much." And so they are likely to conclude: "Therefore, be in control, right, and proper at all times."

Socially, predictable patterns of parenting and environmental conditioning are noted for this personality. The parenting style they experienced could be characterized as both consistent and overcontrolling. As children, they were trained to be overly responsible for their actions and to feel guilty and worthless if they were not obedient, achievement oriented, or "good." The parental injunction to which they were most likely exposed was, "You must do and be better to be worthwhile."

Table 8.3.
Characteristics of Obsessive-Compulsive Personality Disorder

1.	Behavioral appearance	Workaholic/dependable; stubborn/possessive; procrastination/indecisiveness; perfectionistic
2.	Interpersonal behavior	Feeling avoidance; autocratic to peers/ subordinates; obsequious to superiors; polite, loyal
3.	Cognitive style	Constricted—rule based, unimaginative; conflict assertive (defiance) vs. pleasing (obedience)
4.	Feeling style	Grim and cheerless
5.	Parental injunction/ environmental factors	"You must do/be better to be worthwhile." Consistent parental overcontrol. Training in being overresponsible/guilty
6.	Biological/temperament	Anhedonic temperament; first born
7.	Self view	"I'm responsible if something goes wrong." Sees self as reliable, competent, righteous
8.	World view	"Life is unpredictable and expects much. Therefore, be in control, right, and proper."
9.	Self and system perpetuant	Very high expectations (+) harshly rigid behavior and beliefs (+) tendency to be self-critical→rigid rule-based behavior and avoidance of social, professional unacceptability (+) ambivalent behaviors→ reinforcement of obsessive-compulsive style

This obsessive-compulsive pattern is confirmed, reinforced, and perpetuated by the following individual and systems factors: exceedingly high expectations plus harshly rigid behavior and beliefs, along with a tendency to be self-critical, leading to rigid rule-based behavior and the avoidance of social, professional, and moral unacceptability. This, in turn, further reconfirms the harshly rigid behaviors and beliefs of this personality (Sperry & Mosak, 1993).

ASSESSMENT OF OBSESSIVE-COMPULSIVE PERSONALITY DISORDER

Several sources of information are useful in establishing a diagnosis and treatment plan for personality disorders. Observation, collateral information, and psychological testing are important adjuncts to the patient's self-report in the clinical interview. This section briefly describes some characteristic observations that the clinician makes and the nature of individuals. Characteristic response patterns on various objective (i.e., MMPI-2 and MCMI-II) and projective (i.e., Rorschach and TAT) tests are also described.

The obsessive-compulsive's dynamics of circumstantiability, perfectionism, and ambivalence make interviewing these individuals difficult and challenging. Their preoccupation with and focus on details and need for control lead to a seemingly endless struggle about words, issues, and who is in charge, without being able to develop an atmosphere of understanding and cooperation. Open-ended questions confuse them and, instead, they want more focused questions, but interpret them too narrowly. They may bring a notebook of their medical histories, diets, and exercise patterns, or even dreams, expecting to review these details with the clinician. And while they may admit that affects and feelings are associated with these details, they are unwilling to admit the value of expressing those affects, much less talking about them. Their ambivalence is difficult to overcome since they cannot accept assurances that their problems are solvable or that they can tolerate less control in their lives.

The clinician's expression of empathy is problematic for them, since they insist that they are objective and have no feelings. This they are perturbed at the expression of empathy and reject it as irrelevant. They may insist that their problems, not their suffering, are important. Yet, they believe, their problems are unsolvable. The only therapeutic leverage for the clinician is to attempt to get and keep such individuals in touch with their anger and other feelings. But this is difficult as they will attempt to defend or deny affects, and will put forth even more obstructive obsessive thinking to neutralize such therapeutic leverage. Forming a therapeutic alliance obviously is difficult, and the interview often consists of aborted attempts, frustrations, and struggles (Othmer & Othmer, 1989).

The Minnesota Multiphasic Personality Inventory (MMPI-2), the Millon Clinical Multiaxial Inventory (MCMI-II), the Rorschach Psychodiagnostic Test, and the Thematic Apperception Test (TAT) can be useful in diagnosing the compulsive personality disorder, as well as the obsessive-compulsive personality style or trait.

On the MMPI-2, look for a moderately high K (Correction) scale. Since people with obsessive-compulsive features are not inclined to self-disclosure, they seldom leave elevated profiles. However, scales 1 (Hypochondriasis) and 3 (Hysteria) tend to be elevated. If physical complaints are the focus of the distress, scale 1 may be particularly elevated. An elevation on scale 9 (Hypomania) usually reflects the degree to which these individuals are autocratic and dominant in interpersonal relationships. Since scale 7 (Psychasthenia) reflects obsessive-compulsivity, elevation of this scale usually indicates a complaining and querulous attitude (Meyer, 1993).

Expect a high score on scale 7 (Obsessive-Compulsive) on the MCMI-II. Elevations on scale A (Anxiety) are not likely, as these individuals tend to express anxiety somatically. Thus scale H (Somatoform) is likely to be elevated (Choca et al., 1992).

Expect an emphasis on Dd (Unusual Detail) and D (Common Detail) responses on the Rorschach, as well as a high F+% (Form Plus) and fewer W (Whole) and color-based responses. Obsessive-compulsive individuals tend to describe some responses in overly specific detail and to criticize the inkblots (Meyer, 1993).

The TAT stories of these individuals tend to be lengthy, with a variety of the themes. Sometimes the primary theme is lost amid the details of the response; this is particularly likely on cards 2 and 13 MF (Bellak, 1993).

TREATMENT APPROACHES AND INTERVENTIONS

Treatment Considerations

Included in the differential diagnosis of the obsessive-compulsive personality disorder are two other Axis II personality disorders: the dependent personality disorder and the passive-aggressive personality disorder. The most common Axis I syndromes associated with the obsessive-compulsive personality disorder are the social phobia disorder, simple phobias, generalized anxiety disorder, and dysthymia (Turner, Beidel, & Burden, 1991). Other Axis I syndromes are hypochondriasis, somatization disorder, obsessive-compulsive disorder, and psychological factors affecting physical conditions. Occasionally, a brief reactive psychosis may be noted in the decompensated obsessive-compulsive person.

The obsessive-compulsive disorder has a long tradition of treatment, dating back to Freud's case of the Rat Man and Adler's "Case of Mrs. A." Note that it is an Axis I disorder, whereas the obsessive-compulsive personality disorder is an Axis II disorder. As the Rat Man exhibited both Axis I and II disorders, many who have read Freud's account of this case and its treatment have incorrectly assumed that both disorders are the same and are to be treated the same. They are not the same disorder, but in about one third of the cases, both disorders have been shown to be present (Jenike, Baer, & Minichiello, 1990). Baer and Jenike (1992) note that obsessive-compulsive personality disorder is less common in obsessive-compulsive disorder than is dependent, avoidant, or personality disorder not otherwise specified. When both disorders are found together, treatment has been shown to be much more challenging than if only the obsessive-compulsive disorder is present.

INDIVIDUAL PSYCHOTHERAPY

Psychodynamic Psychotherapy Approach

The therapy of obsessive-compulsive patients involves exposing their extreme feelings of insecurity and uncertainty. As they come to identify their neurotic structure as a defense against recognizing those weaknesses, they can begin to develop more adaptive security systems. At the outset of treatment, these patients are unable to abandon their obsessive-compulsive defenses, fearing unspeakable consequences. However, as their esteem grows and awareness of their strengths increases, they are able to take the risks of abandoning these patterns and thus are freer to function more productively. The goal of therapy is to switch from impossible expectations for self and others to more realistic, achievable ones. In short, these individuals come to learn that by relinquishing their rigid, inflexible patterns of control and protection, they can actually feel more productive. Doing psychodynamically oriented psychotherapy with obsessive-compulsive patients requires a number of modifications, primarily involving the clinician's level of activity. The clinician must be active from the beginning through the end of treatment. Clinician passivity, according to Salzman (1980), can lead only to interminable analysis and an atmosphere of confusion. Specifically, free association and a tendency to provide endless details and circumstantiality must be controlled and limited. Because of these patients' need for perfection, they tend to qualify and quantify their descriptions, which confuses and obfuscates. The free-association process tends to defeat its own purpose. Thus the clinician must be active to prevent this tangentiality and distraction by attempting to interrupt the irrelevancies and avoidances. Of course, the major avoidance is affects. Whereas these patients may talk about feelings and emotions, and even about transference and countertransference, they assiduously avoid the expression of affect. The clinician must, therefore, focus on real feelings and their expression, and limit intellectual discussion of affects.

Another modification of traditional analytic methods involves a focus on recent events. Although obsessive-compulsive individuals can discuss anger and hostile behavior associated with past events, they find it very difficult to disclose tender impulses and feelings with regard to recent and here-and-now experiences. Such impulses and feelings are viewed as threatening and dangerous, and Salzman (1980) contends that this is the essence of obsessive-compulsive defenses. It is their failure to express these feelings, rather than their hostile behavior, that initiates retaliatory behavior from others, which in turn inspires their wrath and hostile responses.

Finally, the usual instruction to forego major decisions during the course of therapy must be modified. Because of these patients' fear of making mistakes, such instructions can serve to reinforce their pathological patterns. Instead, risk taking and decision making must be promoted. The techniques for dealing with their indecisiveness are clarification and interpretation of their need for absolutes and certainties. If dream material is utilized, the emphasis must be on the present, and dream content dealt with in the same manner as their other productions.

The goal of treatment is that these individuals achieve some degree of balance and compromise, and instead of needing to be superhuman, be able to function as fallible human persons. Because of their anticipatory anxiety, termination issues abound with these patients. It must be clearly understood by both patients and clinicians that anxiety episodes will occur throughout life, and that continuation in therapy is no guarantee against life's distresses.

A related goal is superego modification so that these patients can accept that their wish to transcend such feelings as anger, lust, and dependency is doomed to failure, and that these feelings must be integrated rather than disowned. Gabbard (1994) notes that such changes occur through detailed interpretation of conflicts around aggression, sexuality, and dependence.

There is a consensus that long-term psychodynamic treatment is needed with these patients, because of their constricted emotionality and their vulnerability to deflation of self-esteem under their rigid exteriors. Treatment of one or two sessions per week typically lasts two to three years. The prevailing wisdom is that dynamic psychotherapy, with the ancillary support of medication and behavioral interventions, is effective (Salzman, 1989).

Cognitive-Behavioral Approach

Beck et al. (1990) provide an extended discussion of the cognitive therapy approach with individuals with obsessive-compulsive personality disorders. The general outcome goal in working therapeutically with these patients is to help them to modify and restructure the maladaptive schemas that underlie their behaviors and affects. Establishing a collaborative working relationship is the first task of therapy. This can be quite difficult for these individuals because of their rigidity, avoidance of feelings, and tendency to minimize the importance of interpersonal relationships. Therefore, rapport is based on the patient's respect for the therapist's competence and the belief that the therapist will be respectful and helpful. Efforts to develop a closer emotional relationship early in treatment may result in premature termination. It is also essential to introduce the obsessive-compulsive individual to the cognitive theory of emotion early in the course of therapy, as well as to establish therapeutic goals. Usually this involves presenting problems. After these goals are collaboratively established, they are ranked in the order in which they are to be addressed. A given problem is monitored between sessions with the dysfunctional thought record, which includes the situation, as well as the person's feelings and thoughts when the problem arose. The record is reviewed at the next session as the basis for discussing automatic thoughts and the assumptions or schemas underlying those thoughts. In this collaborative relationship, the individual can identify and understand the negative consequences of the schemas and ways to refute them. This process of cognitive disputation and restructuring is particularly useful and well received by obsessive-compulsive individuals because of its structured and problem-centered, here-and-now focus.

Several specific strategies and techniques have been found particularly useful with these individuals as adjuncts to cognitive therapy. Setting an agenda, prioritizing problems, and utilizing problem-solving and thought-stopping techniques are effective with issues of rumination, procrastination, and indecisiveness. Salzman (1989) reports that flooding, desensitization, response prevention, and satiation training have been used in treating this disorder. Relaxation training is useful with anxiety and psychosomatic symptoms, and behavioral experiments can be used instead of direct disputation of maladaptive beliefs. Because of the difficulty these persons have in attending to their own emotions and those of others, empathy training and role reversal have been used effectively. In sum, the obsessive-compulsive personality disorder is challenging, but treatable. With collaboration, cognitive restructuring, and the systematic application of cognitive and behavioral strategies and techniques, the obsessive-compulsive individual's automatic thoughts and schemas that underlie the maladaptive behavior and affects can be effectively modified and changed.

Turkat (1990), however, concludes that behavioral modification alone is not sufficient to ensure effective treatment outcomes with most of these patients. His treatment regimen involves social skills training to increase pleasure and emotion-related experiences and to decrease the overcommitment to work. He notes that while these patients would agree with the clinical formulation and treatment plan, most would not agree to undergo the training. Turkat and Maisto (1985) report similar experiences, leading them to conclude that behavior modification alone is not effective for the obsessive-compulsive personality disorder.

Interpersonal Approach

For Benjamin (1993), psychotherapeutic interventions for persons with obsessive-compulsive personality disorders can be planned and evaluated in terms of whether they enhance collaboration, facilitate learning about maladaptive patterns and their roots, block these patterns, enhance the will to change, and effectively encourage new patterns.

Because of the centrality of control in their lives, obsessive-compulsive individuals find collaboration difficult. They are often inconsistent in their attitudes toward control of the therapy, sometimes wanting to take control, and at other times wanting the clinician to take it. Benjamin suggests breaking through a potential power struggle by describing the obsessive-compulsive's typical patterns of control, submission, and self-control and their opposites—affirmation, disclosure, and self-affirmation—and how and why the obsessive-compulsive patterns developed. She notes that these individuals quickly grasp, intellectually, the ideal of friendly differentiation as the opposite of hostile control, and will develop an interest in collaboration. After this shared goal of openness and warmth has been established, they can begin working on experiencing feeling and changing their relational behaviors. Not surprisingly, the work of learning to let go is not easy.

As these individuals begin seeking connections between early life experiences and present difficulties, they must be helped to develop compassion and empathy for themselves as children. Benjamin notes that couples therapy is a particularly potent format for learning about and changing maladaptive patterns in obsessive-compulsive individuals. Dealing with control and power struggles between partners is aided by reframing and paradoxical injunctions. A paradoxical use of their preference for rule following would involve the clinician's "ordering" the obsessive-compulsive patient to collaborate with the partner in developing "rules" for dealing with the problematic relational issues.

Therapeutic efforts to block maladaptive patterns should target power struggles, feeling avoidance, and perfectionism. With regard to perfectionism, undercutting the need to reach perfection through control usually results in reducing anger. As the obsessive-compulsive individual no longer needs to make others perfect, there is no need to be angry with them. This is also true of the anxiety that arises from the fear of not reaching perfection. Since the individual does not need to be perfect to survive, he or she no longer needs to be anxious about not being perfect. As these individuals come to understand the origins of their quest for perfection and to compare their early life situations with the present, they are better able to relinquish their past neurotic strivings. Developing empathy for the self as a child and for the parent at that distant time can strengthen their will to give up their maladaptive patterns.

Cognitive therapy is particularly useful in modifying their constricted cognitive style and self-criticism. Likewise, insight can increase the probability that they will become more comfortable with being fallible and ordinary.

GROUP THERAPY

Because a major deficit of the obsessive-compulsive personality is the inability to share tenderly and spontaneously with others, group treatment has particular advantages with such patients. Nonetheless, there are certain complications, because of these patients' tendency to compete and to try to control situations. Yalom (1985) uses the word "monopolist" to refer to this obsessive-compulsive pattern in group therapy. Such persons can easily dominate a group with their rambling and excessive speech patterns. They may find the affective atmosphere in psychotherapy group overwhelming at first, resulting either in further isolation or in detached intellectualization. The group leader may need to intervene and avoid unnecessary power struggles. If this is achieved, these patients may be able to model vicariously the emotional expressiveness of other group members.

Actually, group therapy offers a number of advantages over individual therapy as the obsessive-compulsive personality pattern tends to make the dyadic-therapy process tedious, difficult, and unrewarding, particularly during the inevitable "constipated" period of treatment when clinicians commonly err with premature interpretations or behavioral prescriptions (Salzman, 1980; Wells, Glickhauf-Hughes, & Buzzel, 1990).

A group format can diffuse the intensity of the patient's impact, particularly in a heterogeneous group (Frances et al., 1984). Group treatment can also reduce transference and countertransference traps because patients are more likely to accept feedback from peers without the power struggle that often accompanies feedback from the clinician (Gabbard, 1994). Furthermore, group therapy propels these patients into having problems rather than just talking about them (Alonso & Rutan, 1984).

Wells and colleagues (1990) note the following contraindications to group therapy for these patients: severe depression or strong suicidal potential, impulsive dyscontrol, strong paranoid propensities, acute crisis, difficulty in establishing trust, fear of relinquishing obsessive-compulsive defenses, the need to establish superiority, and the use of "pseudoinsight" to avoid dealing with both hostile and tender feelings.

These authors describe a unique group approach combining interpersonal and psychodynamic principles that is based on the premise that this personality disorder arises from the unsuccessful resolution of the developmental tasks of autonomy versus shame and doubt. The process of treatment involves six goals: (1) modifying cognitive style, (2) augmenting decision making and action taking, (3) modifying a harsh superego, (4) increasing comfort with emotional expression, (5) resolving control issues, and (6) modifying interpersonal style.

MARITAL/FAMILY THERAPY

The professional literature in this area is particularly limited; however, some of the dynamics and treatments discussed regarding group therapy are relevant in a family treatment context.

Harbir (1981) notes that those with obsessive-compulsive personality disorders typically enter family treatment because close family members are angry with them for their rigidity, procrastination, constricted affect, perfectionism, and somber or joyless outlook. The spouse of an obsessive-compulsive mate may threaten divorce if the individual does not change. Often, such a threat of separation or divorce is the only motivation to seek treatment. With the anxiety of the complaining spouse the only leverage for treatment, the clinician may need to work with that spouse to deal more effectively with the other's obsessive-compulsive personality pattern. Harbir adds that it is not uncommon for an obsessive-compulsive individual to marry an individual with a histrionic personality.

Salzman (1989) cautions that obsessive-compulsive patients who are particularly anxious may not be able to participate in family therapy until their anxiety has been sufficiently ameliorated in individual psychotherapy or combined psychotherapeutic and psychopharmacological treatment. Even when excessive anxiety is not a particular concern, these patients are often tyrants in family sessions. They may immobilize other family members to such an extent that treatment is jeopardized. The use of structural and strategic interventions directed at redistributing power may be advantageous in such situations (Minuchin, 1974).

Regarding treatment outcomes, no controlled research studies have been published. However, Minuchin (1974) and Haley and Hoffman (1967) have reported favorable outcomes with family therapy interventions with obsessive-compulsive personalities, and particularly with those with permanent eating disorders.

Harbir (1981) and Perry, Frances, and Clarkin (1990) present case examples of marital therapy wherein one partner exhibits an obsessive-compulsive personality and the other a histrionic personality. These cases are quite instructive with regard to treatment strategy and techniques.

MEDICATION

No pharmacological trials on the obsessive-compulsive personality disorder per se have been reported, in contrast with the numerous drug studies of obsessive-compulsive disorders. Jenike (1990) reports that cyclic antidepressants, serotonergic blockers, monoamine oxidase inhibitors (MAOIs), lithium carbonate, antipsychotics, and anxiolytics have been effective with obsessive-compulsive disorder, but that medications have little or no effect on obsessive-compulsive personality disorder, and thus psychotherapy is the treatment of choice (Jenike, 1991).

Nevertheless, concurrent Axis I conditions, particularly symptoms of anxiety and depression, may be amenable to medication. Salzman (1989) reports that anxiolytics can relieve coexisting anxiety and that antidepressants can relieve secondary depression.

INTEGRATED AND COMBINED TREATMENT APPROACH

Salzman (1989) elegantly makes the case for a combined/integrated approach to the treatment of the obsessive-compulsive disorder, particularly the more severe cases. He argues that the various treatment modalities and approaches are supplementary rather than mutually exclusive.

Combining treatment should follow a protocol. Since high levels of anxiety or depression may limit participation in psychotherapy, an appropriate medication trial may be useful at the onset of treatment. If rituals or obsessions are prominent, specific behavior interventions—such as response prevention, exposure, habituation, and thought stopping (Salkovskis & Kirk, 1989)—are indicated. The basic dynamics of perfectionism, indecisiveness, and isolation of affect are best attained by psychotherapeutic approaches. Decisions about whether to utilize individual, group, or a marital and family format, or a combination of modalities, are based on the severity of the disorder, the particular treatment target, and specific contraindications. For instance, where isolation of affect and perfectionism are manifest primarily as a rambling speech pattern, an integrative group therapy approach, such as described by Wells et al., (1990), may greatly delimit the resistance and subsequent countertransference so common in dynamic treatment formats. Where indecisiveness is a prominent issue, modeling and other behavioral methods, as well as role playing, might be incorporated into individual treatment formats. In general, the more severe the disorder, the more the treatment needs to be tailored and multimodal.

Salzman (1989) concludes that a true understanding and appreciation of the obsessive-compulsive personality "requires an integration of psychodynamic, pharmacologic, and behavior therapies, because the resolution of the disabling disorder demands cognitive clarity plus behavioral and physiologic alterations. Each modality alone deals with only a piece of the puzzle. A therapist who can combine all these approaches will be the most effective" (Salzman, 1989, p. 2782).

CHAPTER 9

Paranoid Personality Disorder

The paranoid personality disorder is a well-established diagnostic entity. It was listed in the previous versions of the DSM, and references to it are consistently noted throughout the vast literature on schizophrenic and paranoid psychosis. Since Kraeplin's time, the defining feature of the paranoid personality disorder has been a pervasive and unwarranted mistrust and suspiciousness of others. Other clinical features that have been associated with this disorder are hypervigilance, hypersensitivity to criticism, rigidity, and antagonism and aggressiveness. This body of literature formed the basis for the DSM-III criteria, in which patients were required to meet three criteria for suspiciousness, two for restricted affect, and two for hypersensitivity. DSM-III-R was less restrictive, requiring any combination of four of seven criteria (Bernstein, Useda, & Siever, 1993). Only minor changes were made in the DSM-IV criteria, to reduce overlap with other disorders.

Paranoid personality disorder has been described as a paranoid spectrum disorder ranging from the paranoid personality disorder through the delusional disorder to paranoid schizophrenia. The distinguishing feature of the personality disorder is the lack of clear-cut delusions, hallucinations, or other psychotic features. Nevertheless, the boundaries between paranoid personality disorder and delusional disorder, persecutory style, remain unclearly charted (Manschreck, 1992). The psychoanalytic literature also recognized the paranoid personality. Following Freud's formulation, based largely on the Schreber case, analytical writers have related paranoid tendencies to the repudiation of latent homosexuality through projection as the common denominator of this disorder (Akhtar, 1990). Others, like Frosch (1983), contend that the common denominator may be humiliating experiences at the hands of significant others of the same sex, which engendered feelings of having been helpless victims.

The prevalence of this disorder has been estimated at between 0.5 and 2.5 percent in the general population, and in clinical settings, 10 to 30 percent among inpatients and 2 to 10 percent among outpatients.

This chapter describes the characteristic features of the paranoid personality disorder and its related personality style. Five clinical formulations of the disorder and psychological assessment indicators are highlighted. A variety of treatment approaches, modalities, and intervention strategies are also described.

CHARACTERISTICS OF THE PARANOID PERSONALITY STYLE AND DISORDER

The paranoid personality can be thought of as spanning a continuum from healthy to the pathological, with the paranoid personality style at the healthy end and the paranoid personality disorder at the pathological end. Table 9.1 compares and contrasts the paranoid personality style and disorder.

The paranoid personality disorder can be characterized by the following behavioral, interpersonal, cognitive, and emotional styles.

Behaviorally, paranoid individuals resist external influences. They tend to be chronically tense because they are constantly mobilized against perceived threats from their environment. Their behavior also is marked by guardedness, defensiveness, argumentativeness, and litigiousness.

Interpersonally, they tend to be distrustful, secretive, and isolative. They are deeply suspicious of others' motives. They are also intimacy avoiders by nature, and repudiate nurturant overtures by others.

Their cognitive style is characterized by a mistrust of preconceptions. They carefully scrutinize every situation, and scan the environment for "clues" or "evidence" to confirm their preconceptions rather than objectively focus on data. Thus whereas their perceptions may be accurate, their judgment often is not. The paranoid personalities' prejudices mold the perceived data to fit their preconceptions, and they tend to disregard evidence that does not fit. When they are under stress, their thinking can take on a conspiratorial or even delusional flavor. Their hypervigilance and need to seek evidence to confirm their beliefs lead to a rather authoritarian and mistrustful outlook on life.

Table 9.1
Comparison of Paranoid Personality Style and Disorder

Personality Style	Personality Disorder
• Self-assured and confident in their ability to make decisions and take care of themselves.	• Reluctant to confide in others because of unwarranted fear that the information will be used against them.
• Good listeners and observers, keenly aware of subtlety, tone, and multiple levels of meaning.	• Read hidden meanings or threats into benign remarks or events, for example, suspect that neighbors put out trash early to annoy them.
• Take criticism rather seriously without becoming intimidated.	• Bear grudges or are unforgiving of insults or slights.
• Place a high premium on loyalty and fidelity, working hard to earn and maintain them and never taking them for granted.	• Question, without justification, the fidelity of spouses or sexual partners, friends, and associates.
• Careful in dealings with other people, preferring to size up individuals before entering into relationships with them.	• Expect, without sufficient basis, to be exploited or harmed by others.
• Are assertive and can defend themselves without losing control and becoming aggressive.	• Are easily slighted and quick to react with anger or to counterattack.

Their emotional or affective style is characterized as cold, aloof, unemotional, and humorless. In addition, they lack a deep sense of affection, warmth, and sentimentality. Because of their hypersensitivity to real or imagined slights, and their subsequent anger at what they believe to be deceptions and betrayals, they tend to have few, if any, friends. The two emotions they express in some depth are anger and intense jealousy.

The following two cases further illustrate the differences between the paranoid personality disorder (Mr. W.) and the paranoid personality style (Janice L.).

Case Study: Paranoid Personality Disorder

Mr. W., who is 53 years old, was referred for psychiatric evaluation by his attorney to rule out a treatable psychiatric disorder. He had entered into five lawsuits in the past two and one-half years, all of which his attorney believed were of questionable validity. Mr. W. was described as an unemotional, highly controlled man who was now suing a local men's clothing store "for conspiring to deprive me of my consumer rights." He contended that the store manager had consistently issued bad credit reports on him. The consulting psychiatrist elicited other examples of similar concerns. Mr. W. had long distrusted his neighbors across the street, and regularly monitors their activity since one of his garbage cans disappeared two years previously. He took an early retirement from his accounting job one year ago because he could not get along with his supervisor, whom he believed was faulting him about his accounts and paperwork, whereas, he contends, he was faultless. On examination, Mr. W.'s mental status was unremarkable, except for constriction of affect and a certain hesitation and guardedness in his response to questions.

Case Study: Paranoid Personality Style

Janice L. is a 46-year-old tax attorney for a major corporation. Although she had been reluctant to leave her private law practice, the corporation had courted her for several years. They needed a skilled and successful woman to round out their legal team. They made her an offer she could not refuse, and after ensuring that she could maintain sufficient independence in the job, she accepted. Although she had a loose reporting relationship with the chief counsel and two corporate vice-presidents, from the beginning she maintained cordial but somewhat distant relationships with them. She attended only those meetings and social gatherings that were absolutely required. She kept small talk to a minimum, and went about her work with a single-minded vigor that others came to respect, although they could not quite understand her style of relating. When others began to question her standoffish manner, she replied that she had been hired "to be a competent litigator, not a social butterfly." In the courtroom, she was an awesome sight: cool, calm, and collected. She was totally in charge in examining and cross-examining witnesses and in her opening and closing statements. No stone was left unturned and no verbal or nonverbal cue was missed. She instinctively "went to the jugular," as her peers would say, and seldom lost a judgment. There was never a question about her worth or loyalty to the corporation, and in time, her peers and superiors came to accept her unique style.

DSM-IV Description and Criteria

Table 9.2 gives the DSM-IV description and criteria.

Table 9.2
DSM-IV Description and Criteria for Paranoid Personality Disorder[*]

301.0 Paranoid Personality Disorder

A. A pervasive distrust and suspiciousness of others such that their motives are interpreted as malevolent, beginning by early adulthood and present in a variety of contexts, as indicated by four (or more) of the following:

   (1) suspects, without sufficient basis, that others are exploiting, harming, or deceiving him or her

   (2) is preoccupied with unjustified doubts about the loyalty or trustworthiness of friends or associates

   (3) is reluctant to confide in others because of unwarranted fear that the information will be used maliciously against him or her

   (4) reads hidden demeaning or threatening meanings into benign remarks or events

   (5) persistently bears grudges, i.e., is unforgiving of insults, injuries, or slights

   (6) perceives attacks on his or her character or reputation that are not apparent to others and is quick to react angrily or to counterattack

   (7) has recurrent suspicions, without justification, regarding fidelity of spouse or sexual partner

B. Does not occur exclusively during the course of Schizophrenia, a Mood Disorder With Psychotic Features, or another Psychotic Disorder, and is not due to the direct physiological effects of a general medical condition

   Note: If criteria are met prior to the onset of Schizophrenia, add "Premorbid," e.g., "Paranoid Personality Disorder (Premorbid)."

[*]Reprinted with permission from the *Diagnostic and Statistical Manual of Mental Disorders, Fourth Edition.* Copyright 1994 American Psychiatric Association.

FORMULATIONS OF THE PARANOID PERSONALITY DISORDER

Psychodynamic Formulations

Psychoanalytic formulations of the paranoid personality focus on the phenomenon of projection. Essentially, paranoid individuals inaccurately perceive in others that which is true of themselves, and, as by projecting unacceptable feelings and impulses onto these others, experience a reduction of anxiety and distress (Shapiro, 1965).

The self-representation of the paranoid personality involves the coexistence of a special, entitled grandiose self with a weak, worthless, inferior polar opposite (Gabbard, 1990). Developmentally, individuals with paranoid personality disorder are likely to have grown up in an atmosphere charged with criticism, blame, and hostility, and to have identified with a critical parent. Identification with such critical parents suppresses these individuals' feelings of inadequacy and ensures the continuing importance of the mode of criticism in the development and functioning of the personality. Through their identifications, paranoid individuals learn hypervigilance, suspiciousness, and blaming. Hypervigilance and suspiciousness prevent self-criticism, whereas blaming—considered an identification with the aggressor—serves to erase possible experiences of humiliation (Kellerman & Burry, 1989).

Paranoid individuals focus on seeing imperfection in the world around them. This externalization permits a denial of any personal imperfection. Essentially, they feel inferior, weak, and ineffective, and thus grandiosity and specialness are understood as compensatory defenses against feelings of inferiority (Gabbard, 1990).

The primary defense mechanisms of this disorder are projection and projective identification. In addition to externalizing threats with projection, projective identification serves to control others in the environment by binding them in pathological ways. This need to control others reflects a low self-esteem, which is at the heart of the paranoid personality disorder. Basically, it sensitizes these individuals to concerns about all passive surrender to all impulses and to all persons (Shapiro, 1965). Finally, rationalization, reaction formation, and displacement are secondary defense mechanisms.

In short, the need to criticize the world and external objects allows paranoid individuals to maintain an anxiety-free existence in the face of personal imperfections and a grave sense of inadequacy. Profound feelings of inferiority are projected onto the "inferior" world, which is then related to in a consistently critical manner. The self can be then viewed as "good," and "badness" is split off and projected outward.

Cognitive-Behavioral Formulations

From the cognitive therapy perspective, the paranoid personality disorder is characterized by a pattern of certain assumptions, automatic thoughts, and cognitive distortions. Beck et al. (1990) note that individuals with paranoid personality disorders typically view themselves as righteous and as mistreated by others. They tend to see others as interfering, devious, treacherous, covertly manipulative, and discriminatory. They may believe that others form secret coalitions against them. On the basis of this belief that others are against them, these individuals are driven to be hypervigilant and always on guard. They tend to be wary, suspicious, and sensitive to cues that would betray the "hidden motives of their adversaries." When they confront their "adversaries," they often provoke the hostility that they believed already existed. Pretzer (1988) asserts that this attribution of the malicious intent of others is the core assumption of this disorder.

Typical automatic beliefs with this disorder are: "Other people can't be trusted," "People are basically deceptive," "If people act friendly, they are trying to use me," and "If people seem distant, it proves they are unfriendly." Finally, individuals with paranoid personality disorder often utilize the cognitive distortions of dichotomous thinking, selective abstraction, and overgeneralization (Freeman et al., 1990).

Turkat and Maisto (1985), Turkat and Banks (1987), and Turkat (1985, 1986, 1990) have painstakingly studied paranoid personality disorder from the behavioral perspective. Although Turkat (1990) contends that there is no single formulation for this disorder, he notes that hypersensitivity to criticism is usually present. He further notes that such individuals received early training to be frightened at what others think of them, and that they also learned that they are different from others and that they must not make mistakes. As a result of these beliefs, paranoid individuals become overly concerned about and hypersensitive to the evaluations of others and constrained to conform to parental expectations. This, of course, often interferes with acceptance by their peers. Eventually, they are humiliated and ostracized by their peers, partly, because they lack the interpersonal skills necessary to overcome this ostracism. Consequently, they excessively engage in ruminating about their isolation and mistreatment by others. From this, they conclude that the reason for this rejection and persecution is that they are special and others are jealous of them. Accordingly, they act in ways to avoid negative evaluations from others, but these attempts lead them to act differently, which invites social criticism. In their isolation, they brood about their predicament; this engenders persecutory and grandiose thoughts, which further maintain their social isolation. Thus the paranoid patient is caught in a vicious circle that perpetuates the disorder.

Interpersonal Formulation

According to Benjamin (1993), persons diagnosed with paranoid personality disorders were likely to have experienced sadistic, controlling, and degrading parenting. Typically abused children themselves, the parents of paranoid-disordered individuals believed that children are basically evil or bad, require containment, and deserve retribution. Family loyalty was a basic value, and sharing family secrets with others was not tolerated. The adult consequence of such harsh upbringing is that paranoid-disordered individuals expect attack and abuse, even from those close to them. As children, they were harshly punished for dependency, and even attacked when they were sick or hurt or cried. As a result, they learned not to cry, not to ask for help even if injured or sick, and not to trust anyone. As adults, they thus tend to avoid intimacy unless they can control their partners. Often these individuals were subjected to covert as well as overt invidious comparisons within the family, and later among peers. They learned that mistakes and hurts were seldom forgotten, and that grudges were long lasting. Not surprisingly, paranoid individuals are exquisitely sensitive to and angry about exclusion, slights, and even whispering. They tend to be keenly aware of any inequalities in punishments or privileges, and they are likely to sustain grudges for long periods. Furthermore, as children, they were rewarded for competence in helping the family while "staying out of the way." Whereas they were given permission and support to do well, they were degraded and humiliated for venturing out of an assigned area. They came to believe that being a good and lovable person was outside their reach. Subsequently, as adults, they can function competently and independently, but are withdrawn interpersonally. Their expectations of not being acknowledged inspire fear, resentment, and alienation. Finally, they constantly fear that others will attack, blame, or hurt them, while they continue to wish for others to affirm and understand them. Not expecting to be affirmed, they angrily withdraw and tightly control themselves, and if they perceive an attack, will reflexively counterattack.

Biosocial Formulation

In a marked departure from other formulations of the paranoid personality disorder, Millon (1981) and Millon and Everly (1985) conceive of the disorder as a severe form of character pathology. More specifically, Millon and Everly describe it as syndromal continuation of three less severe disorders: narcissistic, antisocial, and compulsive. In their clinical research, they found that individuals with paranoid personalities develop in one of the three syndromal patterns on the basis of their unique biogenic and environmental histories. The narcissistic variation of the paranoid disorder is largely shaped by parental overvaluation and indulgence. As a result, these individuals fail adequately to learn cooperation and interpersonal and responsibility skills. They are often perceived by others as selfish and egotistical. Furthermore, a lack of parental control can give rise to grandiose fantasies of success, power, beauty, or brilliance. In return, they tend to be rejected and humiliated by their peers. These interpersonal rebuffs are followed by increased fantasy and isolation, from which a propensity to paranoia emerges.

The antisocial variant of the paranoid personality exhibits high levels of activation and an impulsive high-energy temperament. The principal environmental determinant seems to be harsh parental treatment. Consequently, these persons develop a deep mistrust of others and exhibit strong self-directedness and arrogance. Because of their tendency to reject both parental and social controls, they also develop aggressive, impulsive, hedonistic lifestyles. Anticipating the attacks of others, paranoid antisocial individuals react irrationally and vindictively. Since they are unable to cope directly with perceived threats, they often erupt in overt hostility.

Individuals with the paranoid-compulsive pattern have developmental histories quite similar to that of the obsessive-compulsive personality disorder. However, their behavior is more irrationally rigid and inflexible (Millon & Everly, 1985). These three versions of the paranoid disorder appear to be self-perpetuated by the individual's own rigidity and suspiciousness. By ascribing slanderous and malevolent motives to others, they remain in a defensive and vindictive posture most of the time. Furthermore, keeping their distance from others allows them to maintain their illusions of superiority, which fosters a self-fulfilling prophesy: as they expect others to be hostile and malevolent, others often become so.

Integrative Formulation

The following integrative formulations may be helpful in understanding how the paranoid personality disorder is likely to develop and be maintained.

Biologically, a low threshold for limbic system stimulation and deficiencies in inhibitory centers seem to influence the behavior of the paranoid personality. The underlying temperament can best be understood in terms of the subtypes of the paranoid disorder. In the narcissistic type, a hyperresponsive temperament and precociousness, parental overvaluation, and indulgence, as well as the individual's sense of grandiosity and self-behavior, probably result in deficits in social interest and limited interpersonal skills. The antisocial type of the paranoid personality is likely to possess a hyperresponsive temperament, which, along with harsh parental treatment, probably contributes to an impulsive, hedonistic, and aggressive style. In the compulsive type, the underlying temperament may have been anhedonia, which, as well as parental rigidity and overcontrol, largely accounts for the development of this type. Finally, a less common variant is the paranoid passive-aggressive type. As infants, these individuals usually demonstrated the "difficult child" temperament, and later a temperament characterized by affective irritability. This, plus parental inconsistency, probably accounts in large part for the development of this type (Millon, 1981).

Psychologically, paranoid individuals view themselves, others, the world, and life's purpose in terms of the following themes. They tend to view themselves by some variant of the theme: "I'm special and different. I'm alone and no one likes me because I'm better than others." Life and the world are viewed by some variant of the theme: "Life is unfair, unpredictable, and demanding. It can and will sneak up and harm you when you are least expecting it." Thus they are likely to conclude: "Therefore, be wary,

Table 9.3
Characteristics of Paranoid Personality Disorder

1.	Behavioral appearance	Guarded and defensive, hypervigilant; resistant to external influences; chronically tense because constantly mobilized against perceived threats; restricted affect, jealous
2.	Interpersonal behavior	Distrustful, secretive, isolated, blaming; provocative, counterattacking, hypersensitive
3.	Cognitive style	Mistrusting of preconceptions—tendency to disregard evidence to the contrary; may become conspiratorial or delusional under stress
4.	Feeling style	Aloof, humorless; easily provoked
5.	Parental injunction/ environment	"You're different. Don't make mistakes." Perfectionistic parent(s) (+) specialness training (+) parental/peer criticalness; isolation (+) vigilant attitude
6.	Biological/temperament	Low threshold for limbic system stimulation and deficient inhibitory centers *Narcissistic type*: hyperresponsive temperament (+) parental overevaluation and indulgence→ deficits in cooperation and interpersonal skills (+) grandiosity/selfishness, aggressiveness *Compulsive type*: anhedonic temperament (+) parental rigidity and control *Passive-aggressive type*: affective irritability (+) parental inconsistency
7	Self view	"I'm so special and different. I'm alone and no one likes me because I'm better than others."
8.	World view	"Life is unfair, unpredictable, and demanding. It will sneak up and harm you. Therefore, be wary, counteract, trust no one, and excuse yourself from failure by blaming others."
9.	Self and system perpetuant	Rigidity and interpersonal suspicion (+) blaming and attributing malevolent motives to others→social alienation and isolation→ confirmation of persecutory stance

counterattack, trust no one, and excuse yourself from failure by blaming others." The most common defensive mechanism associated with the paranoid disorder is projection.

Socially, predictable patterns of parenting and environmental factors can be noted for the paranoid personality disorder. For all of the subtypes, the parental injunction appears to have been, "You're different. Don't make mistakes." Individuals with paranoid personality disorders tend to have had perfectionistic parents who exposed them as children to specialness training. This, plus the parental style that has been articulated for the subtypes of the disorder and parental criticism, leads to an attitude of social isolation and hypervigilant behavior. To make sense of the apparent contradiction between being special and being ridiculed, the children creatively conclude that the reason that they are special and that no one likes them is that they are better than other people. This explanation serves the purpose of reducing their anxiety and allowing them to develop some sense of self and belonging.

This paranoid pattern is confirmed, reinforced, and perpetuated by the following individual and systems factors: a sense of specialness, rigidity, attributing malevolence to others, blaming others, and misinterpreting motives of others, leading to social alienation and isolation, which further confirm the individual's persecutory stance (Sperry & Mosak, 1993).

ASSESSMENT OF PARANOID PERSONALITY DISORDER

Several sources of information are useful in establishing a diagnosis and treatment plan for personality disorders. Observation, collateral information, and psychological testing are important adjuncts to the patient's self-report in the clinical interview. This section briefly describes some characteristic observations that the clinician makes and the nature of the rapport likely to develop in initial encounters with specific personality-disordered individuals. Characteristic response patterns on various objective (i.e., MMPI-2 and MCMI-II) and projective (i.e., Rorschach and TAT) tests are also described.

Interviewing those with a paranoid personality disorder is a delicate challenge. Rapport is hampered by their pervasive belief that others will harm and exploit them. Therefore, they screen all questions for conspirational content and hidden meaning, and assume that any kindness shown by the clinician is a clever maneuver to take advantage of their weakness. Similarly, they cannot allow themselves to relax in the interview, fearful that easing up would make them too vulnerable; thus they justify their suspiciousness and hypervigilance. They can easily confront others, but will not tolerate being confronted. Smooth transitions from topic to topic are essential. Any abruptness may be experienced as an unjustified attempt to trap them, which could lead to anger, counterattack, or termination of the interview (Othmer & Othmer, 1989).

The Minnesota Multiphasic Personality Inventory (MMPI-2), the Millon Clinical Multiaxial Inventory (MCMI-II), the Rorschach Psychodiagnostic Test, and the Thematic Apperception Test (TAT) can be useful in diagnosing the paranoid personality disorder, as well as the paranoid personality style or trait. On the MMPI-2, an elevation on the 6 scale (Paranoia) is common. However, since these individuals tend to be hyperalert about being perceived as paranoid, this scale may be greatly elevated (Turkat, 1990). They are easily irritated by the MMPI's forced-choice format, as well as by the self-disclosure required by many of the items (Meyer, 1993). Scales 3 (Hysteria), 1 (Hypochondriasis), and K (Correction) tend to be high in these individuals, reflecting their use of denial and projection, their inclination to focus on somatic concerns, and their need to present a façade of adequacy.

On the MCMI-II, elevation on scales 6B (Sadistic) and P (Paranoid) are expected. As this personality style often overlaps with the antisocial, the narcissistic, and the passive-aggressive, elevations are likely on scales 6A (Antisocial), 5 (Narcissistic), and 8A (Passive-Aggressive) (Choca et al., 1992).

On the Rorschach, these individuals produce records that are generally constricted, but characterized by more P (Popular) and A (Animal) responses than C (Pure Color) and M (Human Movement) responses. They typically resent ambiguous stimuli, and so respond to the test with condescending criticism, a flipping of cards, and a focus on D (Detail) responses. Occasionally, they reject cards or refuse to continue with the examination (Meyer, 1993).

On the TAT, suspiciousness may characterize their stories. This is particularly likely to occur on cards 9, G, F, 11, and 16 (Bellak, 1993).

TREATMENT APPROACHES AND INTERVENTIONS

Treatment Considerations

Included in the differential diagnosis of the paranoid personality disorder are the following Axis II personality disorders: antisocial personality disorder, narcissistic personality disorder, obsessive-compulsive personality disorder, and passive-aggressive personality disorder. The most common Axis I syndromes associated with the paranoid personality disorder are generalized anxiety disorder, panic disorder, and delusional disorder. If a bipolar disorder is present, an irritable manic presentation is likely. Decompensation into a schizophrenic reaction also is likely. The paranoid and catatonic subtypes of schizophrenia are most commonly noted.

Until recently, the prognosis for the successful treatment of the paranoid personality disorder was guarded. Today, more optimism prevails in achieving these goals of treatment: increasing the benignness of perception and interpretation of reality and increasing trusting behavior. Several treatment strategies and modalities are useful in accomplishing these goals.

INDIVIDUAL PSYCHOTHERAPIES

Psychodynamically Oriented Psychotherapy

Patients with paranoid personalities tend to lead reasonably adaptive and productive lives, and, not surprisingly, are responsive to psychodynamic psychotherapy. Meissner (1978) contends, however, that their treatment is not easy, but requires empathy, patience, and a great deal of sensitivity to their vulnerabilities. He maintains that the treatment process must be slowly paced, with limited, long-term goals. Three treatment principles characterize such treatment (Meissner, 1978, 1986).

First, a meaningful therapeutic alliance must be established and maintained. The therapeutic alliance requires the patient have a certain degree of trust in the clinician, which is difficult for paranoid patients. The clinician's empathic responsiveness and willingness to serve as a container for a range of negative affects is essential. He or she must avoid responding defensively or challenging the patient's perception of events or of the clinician. Instead, the clinician asks for more details and empathizes with the patient's perceptions and affects. Most important, the clinician must resist the countertransference tendency to get rid of undescribable projections by deflecting them back to the patient with premotive interpretations (Epstein, 1984). In short, the patient must come to view the clinician as a benign, disinterested, but friendly helper (Salzman, 1980).

Second, the essential treatment strategy is to convert paranoid manifestations into depression and work through the underlying mourning. The gradual undermining of paranoid defenses and attitudes leads to the emergence of a depressive core in which the patient's inner senses of weakness, defectiveness, vulnerability, and powerlessness come into focus. This is accomplished through counterprojection and "creative doubt" (Meissner, 1986). Depressive elements are worked through in the transference, which allows the patient to begin the process of mourning the frustrated learning and disappointments with early objects.

Third, the clinician must respect the patient's fragile and threatened sense of autonomy and work toward building and reinforcing it in the therapeutic relationship. A commitment to openness, honesty, and confidentiality means that all decisions must be explored with the patient, and that the ultimate choice must be the patient's. This even applies to decisions about medication, when and if they are indicated (Meissner, 1989).

Since these patients tend to be resistant, provocative, and contentious, countertransference issues cannot be underestimated. Behind their defensiveness and arrogance are narcissistic vulnerability, core feelings of shame and humiliation, and a passive longing for dependence. Thus these patients attempt to counter their anxieties by "turning the tables" and making the clinician feel vulnerable, humiliated, and helpless. Clinicians may react with annoyance or impatience, and become confrontative and argumentative. Or they may feel frustrated, discouraged, and victimized. These reactions must be monitored, their impact on therapy analyzed, and efforts initiated to rebalance the therapeutic alliance (Meissner, 1989).

Brief Psychodynamic Psychotherapy
Long-term psychodynamically oriented psychotherapy involves two or more sessions per week for three or more years. However, since patients with paranoid personality disorders do not engage easily in the therapeutic process, they may be reluctant to do such intensive long-term work. On the other hand, receptivity to treatment increases during the crisis period, usually the experience of acute anxiety or depression. Shorter-term therapy that is more crisis oriented might be a preferable way to begin treatment, with such therapy a prelude to longer-term treatment.

Malan (1976) and Balint, Ornstein, and Balint (1972) describe short-term psychotherapy with acute paranoid disorders. Although these treatments were effective with reactive paranoid presentations, this may not be true for the enduring presentations that are more typical of the paranoid personality disorder. There are no published reports of completed successful treatments of the paranoid personality disorder in the context of brief dynamic psychotherapy.

Cognitive -Behavioral Approach

Beck et al. (1990) provide an extended discussion of the cognitive therapy approach with patients with paranoid personality disorders. The initial phase of treatment can be exceedingly stressful for paranoid individuals in that participating in treatment requires self-disclosure, trusting another, and acknowledging weakness, all of which they experience as dangerous. This stress can be reduced by focusing initially on less sensitive issues or by discussing issues directly (i.e., talking about how "some individuals" experience and react to such situations), or by beginning with a more problem-solving approach and behavioral interventions focused on presenting problems. Such strategies, in addition to giving the patients more than the usual amount of control over scheduling appointments or the content of sessions, can facilitate the development of a collaborative working relationship in which they will feel less distrustful and coerced and less need to be vigilant. Trust can be engendered by explicitly acknowledging and accepting the individual's difficulty in trusting the therapist. As this becomes evident and gradually demonstrated through trustworthiness and actions, it provides the evidence on which trust can be based.

A guided discovery approach when working on treatment goals will reveal the manner in which the patient's paranoid pattern contributes to the problems, facilitating collaborative work on his or her distrust of others, feelings of vulnerability, and desire for retribution, rather than the therapist's insisting that these issues be directly addressed. As treatment progresses to working on specific goals, the emphasis should shift to increasing the individual's sense of self-efficacy before attempting to modify interpersonal behaviors, automatic thoughts, or schemas. Developing an increased awareness of another's point of view and learning a more assertive approach to interpersonal conflict are other common treatment goals with these individuals. Traditional cognitive-behavioral techniques such as assertive communication training and behavioral rehearsal are commonly employed to reverse the provocation of hostile reactions from others that previously confirmed paranoid individuals' views of themselves and others.

In instances where hypervigilance and ideas of reference are particularly resistant, the information-processing, social-skills intervention strategy described by Turkat and Maisto (1985) can be exceptionally useful. The goals of treatment are to decrease sensitivity to criticism and modify social behavior. Social skills training consists of instructional role playing, behavioral rehearsal, and videotaped feedback. The patient is taught to attend to more appropriate social stimuli; to interpret that information more accurately; and to receive others' feedback in a nondefensive way and utilize it constructively (Turkat, 1990). Turkat and Maisto (1985) present a detailed case report illustrating these treatment strategies.

Williams (1988) provides a detailed case report of time-limited cognitive therapy with a substance-using depressed college student who also met the criteria for paranoid personality disorder. The patient, who was quite intelligent, was distressed about poor interpersonal relationships and drug use and was motivated for therapy. Noteworthy about Williams's treatment protocol is that only 11 sessions were available, and that these were all that were needed to achieve three treatment goals: to reduce depressive symptoms, to foster less threatening perceptions of the world and other people, and to increase skills in being more relaxed and comfortable with others. Cognitive restructuring and progressive muscle relaxation were the principal intervention strategies. A six-month follow-up showed that all gains had been maintained. Williams concludes that brief cognitive therapy may be particularly well suited for the paranoid personality disorder.

In summary, the cognitive therapy approach to working with paranoid individuals focuses considerable effort on carefully developing a collaborative work relationship and increasing the individual's sense of self-efficacy early in treatment. It utilizes cognitive techniques and behavioral experiments late in therapy to challenge directly the individual's remaining paranoid beliefs.

Interpersonal Approach

For Benjamin (1993), psychotherapeutic interventions with persons with paranoid personality disorders can be planned and evaluated in terms of whether they enhance collaboration, facilitate learning about maladaptive patterns and their roots, block these patterns, enhance the will to change, and effectively encourage new patterns.

Benjamin notes that the major treatment problem with paranoid individuals is establishing a collaborative therapeutic relationship. To the extent that collaboration occurs, paranoia disappears. Accustomed to being abused and humiliated, paranoid individuals view therapists as critical and judgmental, and look for "slip ups," and cues that they want them to leave. Patience and kindness without hints of coercion, criticism, or appeasement are essential for a considerable period during the early stages of therapy.

As treatment proceeds, the patients must learn that their expectations of attack and abusive control stem from past experiences. As such, they can begin appreciating that these expectations are not always appropriate in the present, and that hostility begets hostility. Furthermore, they must come to understand that their defenses of control, avoidance, and anticipatory relationships will elicit attack and alienation in others. Benjamin advocates the use of "verbal holding" as an antidote to their original abuse. Accurate empathy, genuine affirmation of accomplishments, and understanding constitute verbal holding. At the same time, therapists need to confront provocations gently but firmly. Since confrontation is likely to be threatening, therapists must carefully balance it with affirmation. The goal here is proactive criticism, and for these individuals to learn the meaning of feedback and that their feelings of vulnerability and fearfulness do not "prove" that others, including therapists, are attacking them.

Benjamin's discussion of blocking maladaptive patterns in paranoid individuals includes strategies for dealing with various crises, such as aborting or redirecting rageful outbursts at therapists and dealing with homicidal threats and abuse of their children. She believes that honesty, caring, calmness, attentiveness, and a clear commitment to resolving conflicts on the part of therapists are extremely important to paranoid individuals in crisis. Benjamin finds that the wish to relinquish patterns of alienation, hostile control, bearing of grudges, and fearfulness does not develop until these individuals feel it safe to do so. As therapy proceeds, they are helped to lessen their enmeshment with early controlling, attacking figures. As they can see that they are acting like a hated parent, they may become interested in being different.

Once safer bases are established with significant others and with their therapists, they can begin channeling their anger in a direction that encourages separation from earlier destructive patterns and beliefs. Finally, to the extent that therapeutic collaboration develops, considerable new learning about trust, giving and receiving positive and negative feedback, and thinking more benignly about people and life circumstances has already taken place. As these skills are mastered, any residual learning that remains to be acquired by the last stage of therapy is relatively easy to implement. For paranoid individuals at the last stage of treatment, excursions into the social world that further the idea that friendly approaches elicit friendly reactions can be slightly frightening, but also exhilarating.

GROUP THERAPY

Because of their hypersensitivity, suspiciousness, and tendency to misinterpret the comments of others, individuals with paranoid personality disorders tend to avoid group therapy and other forms of group treatment. Similarly, the paranoid tendency to be accusatory, self-righteous, obstinate, hostile, and evasive has been a contraindication to heterogeneous intensive group therapy (Yalom, 1985; Frances et al., 1984; Vinogradov & Yalom, 1989).

Conversely the more highly functioning paranoid patients who can maintain a degree of self-awareness and are able to tolerate a group confrontation of their paranoid distortions may derive considerable benefit from participation in an established group that is sufficiently cohesive and tolerant of divergent opinions (Meissner, 1989).

MARITAL/FAMILY THERAPY

Relatively little has been published on therapy with the paranoid personality per se. Nonetheless, either marital or family treatment can be used alone or concurrently with individual therapy. Meissner (1989) indicates that family therapy might be combined sometime during the course of long-term individual psychotherapy. Such therapy might be indicated for the paranoid adolescent whose family dynamics and interaction patterns interfere with or contribute to the patient's difficulties.

Harbir (1981) details some general principles for couples therapy for the paranoid personality. He notes that paranoid features often lead to severe marital dysfunction. The paranoid person's hypersensitivity, joyless intensity, hypervigilance, extreme mistrust, and jealousy cause considerable suffering for his or her partner—and the nonparanoid partner also causes suffering because his or her actions can exacerbate the paranoid condition. Typically, nonparanoid spouses react passively and secretively when accused or criticized. The more they withdraw and are evasive, the more their paranoid partner becomes suspicious and mistrustful. Therefore, the clinician who is treating a married paranoid patient in individual therapy should consider concurrent couples therapy, or at least a conjoint session with the nonparanoid partner, to modify the marital interaction pattern that seems to be maintaining the psychopathology.

The goal of marital therapy is to enhance the positive growth of the couple by reducing the personality pathology of either or both partners. Harbir (1981) reports that paranoid patients can progress in couples therapy despite the inevitable issues of trust and confidentiality. The clinician needs to be constantly aware of the paranoid partner's close monitoring of the clinician's behavior. These patients invariably become angry if they perceive that the clinician is taking sides, or become jealous of the clinician's relationship with the partner, if the clinician is of the opposite sex. Thus the clinician, just as in individual psychotherapy, must be open and forthright about the specific therapeutic process and rationale. Once a therapeutic alliance has been established, the clinician can support the nonparanoid spouse to confront and challenge the constant mistrust of the paranoid partner. An angry response can be expected at first, but the paranoia will start deceasing. Obviously, such confrontation is only prescribed when the patient has adequate impulsive control and has not been violent.

Harbir describes a detailed case example of conjoint couples therapy involving a paranoid spouse. The treatment involves two stages and illustrates Harbir's therapy approach.

MEDICATION

Until recently, there were little data to support the use of psychotropics for patients with paranoid personality disorders. An open clinical trial utilizing pimozide in an outpatient sample of personality-disordered individuals showed that the antipsychotic greatly improved both the schizoid- and paranoid-personality–disordered subgroups. Methodological problems aside, this study was important in alerting clinicians to a medication whose approved indication is only for Tourette's syndrome (Munro, 1992).

Pimozide is a very selective, postsynaptic antidopaminergic agent that is the consensus drug of choice for delusional disorders (Munro, 1992). Because of the common boundaries between the paranoid spectrum disorders, these various disorders also may have a common pathogenesis (Manschreck, 1992). While awaiting controlled trials of pimozide with patients with paranoid personality disorders and subsequent approval from the Food and Drug Administration, pimozide should be considered only for paranoid patients who exhibit blaming, a low frustration tolerance, and hypersensitivity to criticism.

Fieve (1994) reports that fluoxetine hydrochloride (Prozac) has been very effective in reducing suspiciousness. Fluoxetine is one of several new serotonin reuptake inhibitors that have therapeutic potential for treating a paranoid personality when suspiciousness and irritability are prominent.

COMBINED AND INTEGRATIVE TREATMENT APPROACHES

There are sufficient data to suggest that the paranoid personality disorder no longer is untreatable, as was previously believed, but can be treated successfully. Although treatment with psychodynamic and cognitive-behavioral approaches is considered long term, there has been at least one report of successful time-limited treatment (Williams, 1988). Currently, there are little published data on integrating and tailoring treatment with this disorder. Nevertheless, clinical experience shows that an integrative treatment approach probably can maximize therapeutic outcomes, while decreasing the length of treatment.

In conceptualizing personality disorder as having both temperamental and characterological dimensions, it appears that the dynamic approaches are particularly effective with the characterological dimensions, but are less effective with the temperamental dimensions. It seems that cognitive restructuring and the behavioral information-processing approach (Turkat & Maisto, 1985) are particularly effective in modifying the paranoid's cognitive style of hypervigilance. The cognitive-behavioral approach is also useful with difficulties in relaxing and constricted affects. The interpersonal approach (Benjamin, 1993) seems particularly effective in reducing blame and hypersensitivity to criticism. Thus integrating dynamic, cognitive-behavioral, and interpersonal approaches could have a synergistic effect in changing both the temperamental and characterological dimensions of this disorder. It also appears that combining treatment modalities should increase the efficacy of treatment and its cost effectiveness, especially for the more severe presentations of the disorder. The most obvious combined treatment involves the concurrent or sequential use of family, marital, or group therapy with individual psychotherapy. Also quite promising is the combination of medication (i.e., pimozide or serotonin reuptake inhibitors when they are indicated) with individual psychotherapy.

CHAPTER 10

Schizoid Personality Disorder

The schizoid personality disorder is a member of what has come to be called the "odd cluster" of personality disorders. Coined by Bleuler in 1924, the term described the tendency to turn inward and away from the external world, the absence of emotional expressiveness, the pursuit of vague interests, and simultaneous contradictory dullness and sensitivity. Despite its long clinical and theoretical tradition, schizoid personality was overly inclusive and poorly differentiated in DSM-I and DSM-II, but DSM-III attempted to differentiate it by establishing the diagnoses of avoidant personality disorder and schizotypal personality disorder. The three criteria in DSM-III were sufficiently reflective of much of the preceding descriptive literature. DSM-III-R expanded the criteria to seven, which increased its specificity (Kalus, Bernstein, & Siever, 1993).

However, dynamically oriented clinicians were dissatisfied with DSM-III-R in that the withdrawal of interest in others that had characterized schizoid individuals was apparently a retreat. Schizoid patients may secretly long for close relationships, but assume a defensive posture of detachment because of their fears (Gabbard, 1994). DSM-IV has been somewhat modified to acknowledge these patients' difficulty with enjoying everyday activities.

In epidemiological studies of prevalence, schizoid personality disorder is usually the least commonly diagnosed personality disorder in the general population. Even among the clinical population, its prevalence is only about 1 percent (Stone, 1993).

This chapter describes the characteristic features of the schizoid personality disorder and its related personality style. Five different clinical formulations and several psychological assessment indicators are highlighted. A variety of treatment approaches, modalities, and intervention strategies are described.

CHARACTERISTICS OF THE SCHIZOID PERSONALITY STYLE AND DISORDER

The schizoid personality disorder is characterized by the following behavior and interpersonal, cognitive, and emotional styles.

The behavioral pattern of schizoids can be described as lethargic, inattentive, and occasionally eccentric. They exhibit slow and monotonal speech and are generally nonspontaneous in both their behavior and speech. Interpersonally, they appear to be content to remain socially aloof and alone.

Table 10.1
Comparison of Schizoid Personality Style and Disorder

Personality Style	*Personality Disorder*
• Exhibit little need of companionship, and are most comfortable alone.	• Neither desire nor enjoy close relationships, including being part of a family; have no close friends or confidants (or only one) other than first-degree relatives.
• Tend to be self-contained, not requiring interaction with others in order to enjoy experiences or live their lives.	• Almost always choose solitary activities.
• Even-tempered, dispassionate, calm, unflappable, and rarely sentimental.	• Rarely, if ever, claim or appear to experience strong emotions, such as anger or joy.
• Little driven by sexual needs, and while they can enjoy sex, do not suffer in its absence.	• Little if any desire to have sexual experiences with another person.
• Tend to be unswayed by either praise or criticism and can confidently come to terms with their own behavior.	• Indifferent to the praise and criticism of others; display constricted affects, e.g., are aloof, cold, and rarely reciprocate gestures or facial expressions, such as smiles or nods.

These individuals prefer to engage in solitary pursuits, are reserved and seclusive, and rarely respond to others' feelings and actions. They tend to fade into the social background and appear to others as "cold fish." They do not involve themselves in group or team activities. In short, they appear inept and awkward in social situations.

Their style can be characterized as cognitively distracted; that is, their thinking and communication can easily become derailed through internal or external distraction. This characteristic is noted in clinical interviews when these patients find it difficult to organize their thoughts, are vague, or wander into irrelevance such as discussions of the shoes certain people prefer (Millon, 1981). They seem to have little ability for introspection or to articulate important aspects of interpersonal relationships. Their goals are vague and appear to be indecisive.

Their emotional style is characterized as humorless, cold, aloof, and unemotional. They appear to be indifferent to praise and criticism, and they lack spontaneity. Not surprisingly, their rapport and their ability to empathize with others are poor. In short, they have a constricted range of affective response.

The following case examples further illustrate the differences between the schizoid personality disorder (Mr. Y.) and the schizoid personality style (Mr. P.).

Case Study: Schizoid Personality Disorder

Mr. Y. is a 20-year-old college freshman who met with the director of the introductory psychology course program to arrange an individual assignment in lieu of participation in the small-group research project course requirement. He told the course director that because of a twice-daily two-hour trip between his home and the university, he "wouldn't be available for the research project," and that he "wasn't really interested in psychology and was only taking the course because it was required." Upon further inquiry, Mr. Y. disclosed that he preferred to commute and live at home with his mother, even though he had the financial resources to live on campus. He admitted that he had no close friends or social contacts, and that he preferred being a "loner." He had graduated from high school with a "B" average, but did not date or participate in extracurricular activities, except for the electronics club. He was a computer science major, and "hacking" was his only hobby. Mr. Y.'s affect was somewhat flattened; he appeared to have no sense of humor and failed to respond to attempts by the course director to make contact through humor. There was no indication of a thought or perceptual disorder. The course director arranged for an individual project for this student.

Case Study: Schizoid Personality Style

Mr. P. is a 28-year old, six-year veteran of the U.S. Department of the Interior. He has been a forest ranger since graduating from college. While in school, he excelled in the classroom, but was considered a loner by others. Unlike most of his classmates, he did not pledge a fraternity, because he felt that he really needed to live in a place that was quiet and distraction-free. Mr. P. enjoys his work and has received commendations for it. A year earlier, he was offered a promotion to field supervisor, but turned it down as it would have required him to have regular voice or face-to-face contact with up to 10 forest rangers who would report to him. He had befriended a fellow college student with whom he had roomed for three years and with whom he continues to have occasional contact. He has never considered marriage or a family and so has little interest in dating.

DSM-IV Description and Criteria

Table 10.2 gives the DSM-IV description and criteria.

FORMULATIONS OF SCHIZOID PERSONALITY DISORDER

Psychodynamic Formulations

The inner world of schizoid individuals appears to be different from their outward appearance. Akhtar (1987) describes them as overtly detached, asexual, self-sufficient, and uninteresting, but covertly emotionally needy, exquisitely sensitive and vulnerable, creative, and acutely vigilant. These stark differences represent a splitting or fragmentation of different self-representations that remain integrated. The result is identity diffusion.

Balint (1968) and Nachmani (1984) believe that schizoid individuals' difficulty with relating to others stems from a deficit—inadequate mothering—rather than from an oedipal conflict. In short, these individuals base their decisions to be isolated on the conviction that because they failed to receive maternal nurturance and support as infants, they cannot expect or attempt to receive any emotional supplies from subsequent significant figures. Fairburn (1954) views the isolation of schizoid individuals as a defense against a conflict between a wish to relate to others and a fear that their neediness will harm others. Thus they vacillate between a fear of driving others away by their neediness and a fear that others will smother or consume them. Consequently, all relationships are experienced as dangerous and must be avoided.

Table 10.2
DSM-IV Description and Criteria for Schizoid Personality Disorder*

301.20 Schizoid Personality Disorder

A. A pervasive pattern of detachment from social relationships and a restricted range of expression of emotions in interpersonal settings, beginning by early adulthood and present in a variety of contexts, as indicated by four (or more) of the following:

(1) neither desires nor enjoys close relationships, including being part of a family

(2) almost always chooses solitary activities

(3) has little, if any, interest in having sexual experiences with another person

(4) takes pleasure in few, if any, activities

(5) lacks close friends or confidants other than first-degree relatives

(6) appears indifferent to the praise or criticism of others

(7) shows emotional coldness, detachment, or flattened affectivity

B. Does not occur exclusively during the course of Schizophrenia, a Mood Disorder With Psychotic Features, another Psychotic Disorder, or a Pervasive Developmental Disorder, and is not due to the direct physiological effects of a general medical condition.

Note: If criteria are met prior to the onset of Schizophrenia, add "Premorbid" e.g., "Schizoid Personality Disorder (Premorbid)."

*Reprinted with permission from the *Diagnostic and Statistical Manual of Mental Disorders, Fourth Edition*. Copyright 1994 American Psychiatric Association.

Kellerman and Burry (1989) view this isolation and social distancing as a way of managing anxiety. Schizoid individuals are remote, cool, and aloof, but not necessarily malicious toward others. Typically, schizoid individuals utilize the defenses of repression, suppression, isolation of fantasy affect, displacement, and compensation to ensure distance from others and to avoid anxiety.

Biosocial Formulation

Millon (1981) believes that the schizoid personality is formed by an interaction of biogenic and environmental factors. Millon and Everly (1985) suggest that a proliferation of dopaminergic postsynaptic receptors in limbic and frontal cortical regions accounts for the unusual cognitive activity and inhibited emotional responses of schizoid individuals. Along with this, excessive parasympathetic nervous system dampening could account for their apathy, flattened affect, and underresponsiveness. Finally, Millon and

Everly note that an ectomorphic—thin and frail—body type, which has been associated with shyness and introversion, is common among schizoid individuals.

Major environmental factors involve parental indifferences and fragmented communication patterns. Families of schizoid individuals are typically characterized by interpersonal reserve, formality, superficiality, and coldness. They tend to communicate in a fragmented, aborted, and circumstantial fashion. Not surprisingly, individuals raised in such environments are likely to be vague, abortive, and circumstantial in all of their communications. These disjointed communication patterns tend to be confusing to others and to foster their misunderstanding, frustration, lack of tolerance, and hostility. Schizoid individuals are prone to be isolative and come to believe that others do not understand them. Furthermore, they are usually incapable of correcting the problem.

The schizoid disorder is perpetuated by social distancing, by having the social isolation reinforced, and by cognitive and social insensitivity. The infrequent social activities of such individuals limit their ability to grow, and their social isolation is frequently reinforced by others, who ostracize isolative individuals. Furthermore, their social and cognitive insensitivities tend to oversimplify and make boring a world that is so rich and diverse for others.

Cognitive-Behavioral Formulations

From the cognitive therapy perspective, the schizoid personalty is characterized by a pattern of certain assumptions, automatic thoughts, and cognitive distortions. The basic assumptions of schizoid individuals involves their views of self and others. They tend to see themselves as loners and self-sufficient, and the world and others as intrusive. Their core beliefs include: "I am basically alone," and "Relationships are messy and undesirable because they interfere with my freedom of action." Subsequently, their primary interpersonal strategy is to distance themselves from others.

Beck et al. (1990) note that schizoid individuals find it difficult to identify automatic beliefs, probably because emotions are related to thoughts and schizoids have limited emotions. Nonetheless, their automatic thoughts reflect their preference for solitude and their perceptions of being detached observers of life: "I'd rather do it myself," "I prefer to be alone," and "Keep your distance." Finally, neither Freeman et al. (1990) nor Beck et al. (1990) describe cognitive distortions unique to the schizoid personality.

From the behavioral perspective, neither Turkat and Maisto (1985) nor Turkat (1990) offer a formulation for this disorder. They admit interviewing individuals who met the criteria for the disorder, but are unable to offer a generic behavioral formulation.

Interpersonal Formulation

According to Benjamin (1993), persons diagnosed with schizoid personality disorders were likely to have been raised in a home that was orderly and formal. Although their physical and educational needs were met, there was little warmth, play, or social and emotional interaction within the family or elsewhere. The schizoid individual would have modeled social isolation and colorless, unemotional functioning. Such identification with withdrawn parents leads schizoid individuals to expect little and to give little. Although they may be socialized for work, they are not predisposed to intimate contact, and prefer fantasy and solitary advocating. In short, they have neither fears of nor desires about others. Underdeveloped in social awareness and skills, they can meet social role expectations as employees, or even as parents. They may be married, but do not develop close, intimate relationships.

Integrative Formulations

The following integrative formulation may be helpful in understanding how the schizoid personality develops and is maintained.

Biologically, the schizoid personality is likely to have had a passive and anhedonic infantile pattern and temperament. Millon (1981) suggests that this pattern results, in part, from increased dopaminergic postsynaptic limbic and frontal lobe receptor activity. Constitutionally, the schizoid is likely to be characterized by an ectomorphic body type (Sheldon & Stevens, 1942).

Psychologically, schizoids view themselves, others, the world, and life's purpose in terms of the following themes. They view themselves by some variant of the theme: "I'm a misfit from life, so I don't need anybody. I am indifferent to everything." For schizoid personalities, the world and others are viewed by some variant of the theme: "Life is a difficult place and relating to people can be harmful." As such, they are likely to conclude: "Therefore, trust nothing and keep a distance from others and you won't get hurt." Adler (1956) and Slavik, Sperry, and Carlson (1993) further describe these life-style dynamics. The most common defense mechanism utilized is intellectualization.

Socially, predictable patterns of parenting and environmental factors can be noted for schizoids. The parenting style was usually characterized by indifference and impoverishment. It is as if the parental injunction was: "You're a misfit," or "Who are you, what do you want?" Their family patterns are characterized by fragmented communications and rigid, unemotional responsiveness. Because of these conditions, schizoids are grossly undersocialized and develop few, if any, interpersonal relating and coping

Table 10.3
Characteristics of Schizoid Personality Disorder

1.	Behavioral appearance	Speech is slow and monotonous; lethargic, inattentive, nonspontaneous
2.	Interpersonal behavior	Minimal "human" interests and friends; "cold fish" fades into social background; rarely responds to feelings or actions of others, isolated; content to remain aloof
3.	Cognitive style	Cognitively distracted—thoughts and communications are easily derailed and tangential or loose, absentminded; minimally introspective; defense is intellectualization
4.	Feeling style	Aloof, indifferent
5.	Parental injunction/ environmental factors	"Who are you, what do you want?" Rigid, emotionally unresponsive family of origin; fragmented family communications; under-socialized in interpersonal skills
6.	Biological/temperament	Passive and anhedonic infantile pattern; excessive dopaminergic postsynaptic limbic and frontal lobe receptors; ectomorphic build
7.	Self view	"I'm a misfit from life, so I don't need anybody." "I'm indifferent to everything."
8.	World view	"Life is a difficult place and can be harmful. Therefore, trust nothing and keep your distance from others and you won't get hurt."
9.	Self and system perpetuant	Infrequent social activity (+) social insensitivity→reinforcement of social isolation and schizoid style

skills. This schizoid pattern is confirmed, reinforced, and perpetuated by the following individual and systems factors: Believing themselves to be misfits, they shun social activity. This, plus social insensitivity, leads to reinforcement of social isolation and further confirmation of the schizoid style (Sperry & Mosak, 1993).

ASSESSMENT OF SCHIZOID PERSONALITY DISORDER

Several sources of information are useful in establishing a diagnosis and treatment plan for personality disorders. Observation, collateral information, and psychological testing are important adjuncts to the patient's self-report in the clinical interview.

This section briefly describes some characteristic observations that the clinician makes and the nature of the rapport likely to develop in initial encounters with specific personality-disordered individuals. Characteristic response patterns on various objective (i.e., MMPI-2 and MCMI-II) and projective (i.e., Rorschach and TAT) tests are also described.

Interviewing individuals with schizoid personality disorders can seem an exercise in futility given their pervasive emotional withdrawal. They express little or no emotionality, even when talking about anxious or depressed feelings. More intelligent persons with this disorder may complain about anhedonia, and even may use the label "depression," but seldom report associated sadness or guilt. Since emotional warmth is absent, it is difficult to judge whether problems or concerns are central to them. Typically, they have one-word or short-phrase answers to all questions. Neither open-ended questions, structured questions, nor other interview strategies will change the flow of information or expression of affect. Unlike paranoid individuals, this restricted verbal and emotional expression is not due to self-protectiveness, but to emotional and mental emptiness. Rapport usually reflects a willingness to reveal symptoms, problems, and innermost feelings. Since these patients are so impoverished, rapport and engagement may seem impossible. Long periods of silence are not uncommon. If they return for sessions, it usually means that they are "connecting" as much as they know how. Thus the clinician's persistence, patience, and tolerance for limited verbal interchange may have a therapeutic effect (Othmer & Othmer, 1989).

The Minnesota Multiphasic Personality Inventory (MMPI-2), the Millon Clinical Multiaxial Inventory (MCMI-II), the Rorschach Psychodiagnostic Test, and the Thematic Apperception Test (TAT) can be useful in diagnosing the schizoid personality disorder, as well as the schizoid personality style or trait. On the MMPI-2, a normal profile is common for reasonably well-integrated schizoid individuals. In such instances, O (Social Introversion) may be elevated (Lachar, 1974). As they become distressed, rises in F (Frequency), 2 (Depression), and 8 (Schizophrenia) are likely. Occasionally, a 1-8 (Hypochondriasis–Schizophrenia) "nomadic" profile is noted wherein interpersonal attraction is limited.

On the MCMI-II, an elevation on scale 1 (Schizoid) with low scores on 4 (Histrionic), 5 (Narcissistic), and N (Bipolar–Manic) are likely (Choca et al., 1992).

On the Rorschach, a high percentage of A (Animal) and few C (Color) responses are likely. The overall record tends to be constricted and certain blots may be rejected. The reaction times to many of the cards may be slow. There may be a higher experience potential than experience actual and their M (Human Movement) production will be high relative to the overall quality of the protocol (Exner, 1986).

On the TAT, constricted response, along with a blindness of theme, is common, as is an impoverished portrayal of story characters (Bellak, 1993).

TREATMENT APPROACHES AND INTERVENTIONS

Treatment Considerations

Included in the differential diagnosis of the schizoid personality disorder are the following Axis II personality disorders: avoidant personality disorder, schizotypal personality disorder, and the dependent personality disorder. The most common Axis I syndromes likely to be associated with the schizoid personality disorder are depersonalization disorder, the bipolar and unipolar disorders, obsessive-compulsive disorder, hypochondriasis, schizophreniform, and disorganized and catatonic schizophrenias.

Schizoid personalities rarely volunteer to be treated unless decompensation is present. However, they may accept treatment if someone, such as a family member, demands it.

INDIVIDUAL PSYCHOTHERAPY

Some form of individual psychotherapy is indicated for the majority of schizoid patients. Whether the clinician chooses an active confrontative approach, a cognitive restructuring and social skills training approach, or an approach that is more supportive depends on a number of factors, including the patient's psychological mindedness, resilience, and treatment expectations; the clinician's therapeutic repertoire; and resources for treatment.

This section briefly describes the psychodynamic, cognitive-behavioral, and interpersonal approaches to individual therapy.

Psychodynamically Oriented Psychotherapy Approaches

Because the dynamic understanding of both the schizoid and schizotypal personality are inherently similar, Gabbard (1990, 1994) proposes that their treatment is similar. Schizoid patients can be treated effectively with dynamically oriented psychotherapy, both expressive and supportive, depending on their level of functioning and treatment readiness (Gabbard, 1994). The basis for dynamic treatment is not interpretation of conflict, but rather internalization of a therapeutic relationship (Stone, 1985).

Essentially, the clinician's task is to meet the patient's frozen internal object relations by providing a correct emotional experience. The schizoid's style of relatedness results from inadequacies in early relationships with parental figures. As a result, these patients go through life distancing themselves from others. Therapy thus must provide a new relationship for internalization (Gabbard, 1994).

Since their basic mode of functioning is nonrelational, they find the task of therapy very challenging and difficult. Not surprisingly, they respond to the challenge with silence and emotional distancing. Clinicians need to adopt a permissive, accepting attitude, and must be exceedingly patient with these individuals. It is more helpful to understand silence as a nonverbal form of relating than as treatment resistance. By listening with a third ear, the clinician can learn much about these patients. Through projective identification, they will evoke certain responses in the clinician that contain valuable diagnostic information regarding the patient's inner world (Gabbard, 1989). Dealing effectively with countertransference issues is critical in working with schizoid patients. Accepting silent nonrelatedness is foreign to the clinician's psychological predisposition and training, and so, when silence is prolonged, he or she must guard against acting out and projecting his or her own self and object representations onto the patient. Accepting the silence, and refraining from interpreting it, legitimizes the patient's private, noncommunicative core self. And it may be the only viable technique for building a therapeutic alliance (Gabbard, 1989).

The proper pace and depth of therapy are controversial. Bonime (1959) advocates an active, confrontative approach, whereas Gabbard (1990) and others maintain that a more restrained approach is more respectful and less threatening for these patients.

Supportive techniques can be utilized to encourage the lower functioning schizoid to become more active. For example, the patient is first urged to engage in activities where others are present, but where the patient's participation is minimal, as at a sports event. If some level of comfort is achieved, further involvement may be encouraged. Involvement in a computer club, travel tour, or aerobics class is more risky than attending a sporting event, but less risky than a social gathering or a dance class. Kantor (1992) advocates using "productive substitution" and "modification total push" with these therapeutic tasks. In productive substitution, the clinician suggests gratifying replacements for what is missing from the patient's life. Thus relationships with peers in a therapy group substitute for spousal relationships for unmarried patients. Using modified total push, the clinician urges the patient to become more active socially. Suggestions are presented tentatively to test the patient's limits. Problems encountered are brought back into therapy and discussed. Treatment goals and outcomes may be quite limited: the patient may eventually work, but in isolation, that is, as a night watchman; may have one or two social friends; and may even have a long-term relationship with someone who is willing to remain a distant companion (Kantor, 1992).

Long-Term Versus Short-Term Dynamic Therapy

Decisions about the type and frequency of dynamic therapy should be based on the patient's level of functioning and motivation and readiness for treatment. More highly functioning schizoid patients who exhibit some depressive symptoms or some capacity for empathy and emotional warmth tend to have better outcomes in dynamic psychotherapy (Stone, 1985, 1989a).

Those patients who are highly motivated for exploratory psychotherapy can make dramatic gains in intense, long-term treatment of two to three sessions per week over several years. On the other hand, long-term supportive psychotherapy is indicated for the majority of schizotypal patients who present with major ego deficits and personal eccentricities. The goal of such treatment is improved adaptive functioning in day-to-day living. The frequency of sessions is one to two times per week for most patients (Stone, 1989a).

Short-term dynamic therapy is indicated for crisis issues and situational difficulties related to the patient's job or personal life. It may also serve as follow-up to a previous course of long-term psychotherapy. There are no reports of short-term dynamic individual treatments as curative interventions.

Cognitive-Behavioral Approach

Beck et al. (1990) describe the cognitive therapy approach to working with individuals with schizoid personality disorders. As schizoid individuals tend to have limited motivations for social interaction, a principal treatment goal is to establish or increase positions of social interaction, as well as to reduce social isolation. These individuals enter treatment largely because of symptomatic Axis I disorders rather than to alter their manner of relating to others. Thus the initial goal of treatment is a collaborative focus on presenting problems. As this occurs, the therapist can comment on the individual's relational patterns, discussing their advantages and disadvantages, and how they affect the presenting problem. The collaborative therapeutic relationship can itself be a prototype for other interpersonal relationships, as well as a basis for increasing the individual's range and frequency of interactions outside sessions. After rapport has been established, the therapist can point out the characteristic interaction patterns, as well as give feedback on how they affect other persons. As these individuals develop a greater awareness and understanding of interpersonal relating, they are guided in learning needed social skills and practicing them both within and outside of the sessions. Given their lack of expressiveness, routinely soliciting feedback on their level of anxiety should reduce the likelihood of premature termination. Unlike work with other personality disorders where considerable therapeutic leverage and motivation for change are available, relatively little of either is likely with schizoid individuals other than reason. Accordingly, Freeman et al. (1990) advise therapists to clearly present the rationale for therapy, the reasons for acting differently, the advantages and disadvantages of changing behavior, and the concrete gains possible. Presumably, this strategy can induce these individuals to change.

Beck et al. (1990) indicate that the following techniques are effective with schizoid individuals. The dysfunctional thought record not only is useful in challenging dysfunctional automatic thoughts, but also in identifying a variety of affects and their subtle gradation in intensity, as well as indicating the reactions of others. Teaching social skills is best done directly through role playing, in vivo exposure, and homework assignments. Helping these individuals to become more attentive to and to experience positive emotions can be facilitated by guided discovery. For example, as they are helped to recognize their overgeneralized view of others ("I don't like people"), they can learn to be specific about the things they really do not like, as well as those they do like, about others after all.

As treatment nears termination, the matter of relapse prevention is discussed. Beck et al. (1990) report that schizoid individuals are likely to relapse into a isolative lifestyle after termination. Thus they suggest maintaining contact with them through booster sessions. Finally, although treatment with these individuals can be difficult, with persistence it is possible to improve their social skills and frequency of social interaction and to decrease their "strangeness." However, the therapist should anticipate that schizoid individuals are likely to retain some distance and passivity in interpersonal relations even after planned termination.

Interpersonal Approaches

Benjamin (1993) provides no discussion of treatment goals or strategies for the schizoid personality disorder.

GROUP THERAPY

Schizoid patients can profit from group therapy, particularly dynamic group therapy (Azima, 1983). Group therapy offers these patients a socialization experience involving exposure to and feedback from others in a safe, controlled environment. It is an environment in which new parenting can occur. Here, group members can function as a reconstructed family and provide a corrective emotional experience that can counterbalance the schizoid's negative and frightening internal objects (Appel, 1974). As their worst fears are not realized and they feel accepted, these patients gradually become more comfortable with others.

From an object relations perspective, Leszcz (1989) contends that the group functions as a holding environment that provides an opportunity for these patients to become initially involved in a "nonrelating" way while slowly building trust. They do not have to leave their cocoon of self-sufficiency, but can observe how others relate in the groups, how feelings make a difference, and how to deal with negative affects. The wise group leader will permit this nonrelated position until the patient is better able to tolerate the ambiguities of the group.

From a systems perspective, Bogdanoff and Elbaum (1978) maintain that the schizoid's isolation is not simply the result of a fragile ego, but is also a function of the group's need to maintain that isolation. Thus whereas the schizoid patient may provoke the group to make him or her speak, at other times, the group effectively silences the schizoid frightening him or her by rage or blaming. Essentially, the schizoid is caught in an interpersonal trap—which is called a "role lock." Successful group interaction can occur only when the role lock is broken. If the group is avoiding the schizoid, the therapeutic task is to focus the group's attention on the role lock. The aim is for group members to reveal their contribution to the lock and to relieve pressure on the locked member, and for the locked member to reveal how he or she sees the group process to isolate himself or herself.

From an interpersonal perspective, Yalom (1985) discusses other useful interventions for dealing with role lock. Schizoids are helped to differentiate responses to different group members, to take seriously feelings in the here-and-now, and to become more aware of their specific avoidance strategies and their bodily responses. Yalom insists that these goals and strategies are preferable to cathartic methods, which can drive the schizoid from the group. He cautions that the process is slow and that patience is essential for the clinician.

Finally, there seems to be a consensus of sorts that heterogeneous groups are preferable to homogeneous groups (Leszcz, 1989; Bogdanoff & Elbaum, 1978; Slavik, Sperry & Carlson, 1992). Spotnitz (1975) suggests that the schizoid patient be referred to a group that is homogeneous in terms of global functioning, but heterogeneous in terms of personality types.

MARITAL AND FAMILY THERAPY

Schizoid patients, particularly men, do not marry and seldom become self-supporting. They may reside with and become dependent on their families. This can result in a vicious circle in which limited motivations for social contacts and a job or career lead to interference and bitterness on the part of the family, which is followed by lowered self-esteem and an even greater reluctance to leave home (Stone, 1989a).

Clinicians working with schizoid patients still living at home often confront family tension, impatience, and discord arising from differences between parental expectations and the patient's capacities and motivation. Family therapy can be quite effective in addressing these expectational differences, discord, and impatience (Anderson, 1983). Shapiro (1982) describes how the family therapist can function to contain such displaced and projected affects and impulses, and to acknowledge, bear, work through, and redirect them. Family treatment also can help family members to reestablish more functional communication patterns between themselves and the patient.

McCormack (1989) describes a common marital constellation in which schizoid individuals marry borderline individuals. In discussing the treatment of the schizoid spouse, McCormack indicates that the core of the schizoid's difficulty is an overwhelming fear of attachment. Insecurity arises from escalating aggression because frustration of their dependency needs leads to marital dissatisfaction and discord. Schizoid spouses experience their love as lethal, and then abort awareness of these feelings and dependency needs as a defense against them. Thus they develop and maintain relationships in which they are never fully involved.

The treatment of schizoid spouses emphasizes clarification and careful interpretation and deemphasizes confrontation. Exploration should involve their narcissistic vulnerability, legitimization of their needs, acknowledgment of the potential risks and gains attached to pursuing them, and the schizoid compromise. McCormack describes the "schizoid compromise" as a means of maintaining relationships that require limited emotional involvement at the cost of limiting personality development. The clinician needs to acknowledge to these patients that this compromise has been adaptive, but is a stage through which they must pass before facing their fear of genuine, healthy relationships.

Schizoid spouses tend to treat others as they fear being treated, which is frustrating for those who want to have an intimate relationship with them. In conjoint sessions, the clinician helps both spouses to see that each suffers from difficulties that are both similar to and different from their own, and that though these difficulties are fostered in the marriage relationship, they also exist independently of it.

Couples therapy with the schizoid–borderline relationship may require the referral of one spouse for individual therapy, the use of medication, or hospitalization. Long-term couples' treatment is usually necessary if the goal is to foster separation and autonomy, increased marital satisfaction, and harmony.

MEDICATION

Stone (1989a) notes that schizoid patients show such target symptoms as anxiety and depression for which common psychotropic agents are indicated. However, their basic temperamental traits of aloofness and uncommunicativeness tend to make them nonresponsive to current medications.

Because of its apparent overlap with avoidant personality disorder and schizotypal disorder, Liebowitz et al. (1986) suggest that the clinician consider two potential target symptoms for pharmacotherapy. Because hypersensitivity to rejection and criticism—a criterion for the avoidant disorder—may be related to the schizoid patient's social isolation and aloofness, a trial of a monoamine oxidase inhibitor (MAOI) or serotonin reuptake blocker has some efficacy with this target symptom. Fluoxetine (Coccaro, 1993) is another choice. Furthermore, because the schizoid and schizotypal personality disorders lie on the schizophrenic spectrum, and because low-dose antipsychotics have had some efficacy with mixed personality disorder groups that included schizoid patients (Reyntjens, 1972; Barnes, 1977), they may have some place in the treatment of the schizoid personality (Liebowitz et al., 1986).

COMBINED AND INTEGRATED TREATMENT APPROACHES

Schizoid patients tend to avoid mental health professionals just as they avoid relationships in general. When they do present for help, often at the urging of their families, they tend to terminate therapy prematurely after a short time (Stone, 1989a). This means that there is only a small window of opportunity to engage these patients in the therapeutic process. Combining treatment modalities and integrating treatment approaches can facilitate both commitment to treatment and positive treatment outcomes.

Gabbard (1994) advocates combining dynamic group therapy with dynamic individual psychotherapy as the treatment of choice for the majority of schizoid patients. However, he cautions, many of these patients will recoil at the recommendation for group therapy, and may even feel betrayed by their clinician. Thus Gabbard suggests that before making a group referral, fantasies about the group experience need to be explored and worked through. Stone (1989a) also recommends combining individual and group modalities. However, he proposes a developmental approach in which the patient first forms a stable dyadic relationship with the clinician and then proceeds to group therapy with the same clinician. In both instances, the combined treatment is concurrent.

As noted earlier, McCormack (1989) makes the case for combining marital therapy with individual therapy, particularly when there are considerable splitting and projective identification. Combining family therapy and individual therapy has advantages, particularly if the schizoid patient is dependent on the family financially and/or resides with the family. Family can greatly influence the patient's continuation in individual and/or group treatment.

Slavik, Sperry and Carlson (1992) advocate both combining treatment modalities and integrating treatment approaches. They indicate the utility of concurrent individual and group treatment. They also describe how an Adlerian approach can be integrated with an object-relations-theory approach, social skills training, hypnosis, and psychodrama, depending on the patient's style, needs, and expectations. These authors believe that the schizoid personality disorder is eminently treatable, and that these patients have largely gone untreated because clinicians have not found enough ways to engage and encourage them in the change process.

CHAPTER 11

Schizotypal Personality Disorder

Schizotypal personality disorder is part of the "odd" cluster of DSM-IV personality disorders. It was the first of the personality disorders to be defined owing to its genetic relationship to schizophrenia. The genesis of this disorder came from concerns of a DSM-III committee that the definitions of borderline and schizoid personality disorders were too broad and diffuse. The borderline disorder originally was to include both affective instability and schizophrenic-like symptoms. Similarly, the schizoid personality was broadly defined as characterizing individuals with enduring psychotic-like traits. As a result, the schizotypal personality disorder was designated as distinct from both borderline and schizoid personality disorders. DSM-III designated eight criteria. Essentially, the only change in DSM-III-R was to add another criterion: odd and eccentric behavior or appearance. Considerable controversy about the overlap between schizotypal and avoidant personality disorder regarding interpersonal relations was engendered by both DSM-III and DSM-III-R criteria. Between the appearance of DSM-III-R and DSM-IV, compelling evidence was found that demonstrated a link between schizotypal personality disorder and schizophrenia in terms of phenomenological, genetic, biological, outcome, and treatment-response characteristics. As a result, serious consideration was given to shifting the diagnosis from Axis II to the Axis I category of schizophrenia and other psychotic disorders (Siever, Bernstein, & Silverman, 1991). However, the disorder has remained in Axis II of DSM-IV, but with a significant modification of the criteria. Now, psychotic-like symptoms must be persistent rather than episodic as in the borderline personality disorder. Furthermore, the qualification that severe social anxiety does not decrease with familiarity further distinguished it from avoidant personality. But despite changes in the DSM-IV criteria, many psychodynamically oriented clinicians are not convinced that schizoid and schizotypal personality disorders are really different, and consider them inherently similar (Gabbard, 1994).

Prevalence data show that this disorder occurs in 3 percent of the general population. There are no current data on its prevalence in the clinical population.

This chapter describes the characteristic features of the schizotypal personality disorder and its related style. Five clinical formulations of the disorder and psychological assessment indicators are highlighted. A variety of treatment approaches, modalities, and intervention strategies are also described.

CHARACTERISTICS OF SCHIZOTYPAL PERSONALITY STYLE AND DISORDER

The schizotypal personality can be thought of as spanning a continuum from healthy to pathological, where the schizotypal personality style is closer to the healthy end and the schizotypal personality is at the pathological end. Table 11.1 compares and contrasts the schizotypal personality style and disorder.

The schizotypal personality disorder typically is recognized by the following behavioral, interpersonal, cognitive, and affective or emotional styles.

Behaviorally, schizotypals are noted for their eccentric, erratic, and bizarre mode of functioning. Their speech is markedly peculiar without being incoherent. Occupationally, they are inadequate, either quitting or being fired from jobs within short periods of time. Typically, they become drifters, moving from job to job and from town to town. They tend to avoid enduring responsibilities and in the process lose touch with a sense of social propriety.

Interpersonally, they are loners with few, if any, friends. Their solitary pursuits and social isolation may be the result of intense social anxiety. This may be expressed by apprehensiveness, which does not diminish with familiarity, and is associated with paranoid features rather than negative self-appraisal. If married, their style of superficial and peripheral relating often leads to separation and divorce in a relatively short time. Their lives

Table 11.1
Comparison of Schizotypal Personality Style and Disorder

Personality Style	*Personality Disorder*
• Tend to be tuned into and sustained by their own feelings and belief affects.	• Have ideas of reference; suspicious or paranoid ideation; inappropriate or constricted affect.
• Are keenly observant of others and particularly sensitive to how others react to them.	• Have excessive society anxiety, e.g., extreme discomfort in social situations involving unfamiliar people.
• Tend to be drawn to abstract and speculative thinking.	• Have odd beliefs or magical thinking that influences behavior and is inconsistent with subculture norms, e.g., superstition, belief in clairvoyance, telepathy, or a "sixth sense," and that others can feel their feelings.
• Are receptive to and interested in the occult, the extrasensory, and the supernatural.	• Have unusual perceptual experiences, e.g., illusions, sensing the presence of a force or person not actually there (e.g., "I felt as if my dead mother were in the room with me").
• Tend to be indifferent to social convention, and have interesting and unusual life-styles.	• Are odd or eccentric in behavior or appearance, e.g., unkempt, unusual mannerisms, talk to self; odd speech (without loosening of association) or incoherent, e.g., speech that is impoverished, digressive, vague, or inappropriately abstract.
• Usually are self-directed and independent, requiring few close relationships.	• Have no close friends or confidants (or only one) other than first-degree relatives.

tend to be marginal, and they gravitate toward jobs that are below their capacity or demand little interaction with others.

The cognitive style of schizotypals is described as scattered and ruminative, and is characterized by cognitive slippage, including presentations of superstition, telepathy, and bizarre fantasies. They may describe vague ideas of reference and recurrent illusions of depersonalizing, derealizing experiences without the experience of delusions of reference or auditory or visual hallucinations.

Their affective style is described as cold, aloof, and unemotional, with constricted affect. They can be humorless and difficult to engage in conversation, probably because of their general suspicious and mistrustful nature. In addition, they are hypersensitive to real or imagined slights.

The following two case examples further illustrate the differences between the schizotypal personality disorder (Ms. S.) and the schizotypal personality style (Mr. P.).

Case Study: Schizotypal Personality Disorder

Ms. S., a 41-year-old single woman, was referred to a community mental health clinic by her mother because she had no interests, friends, or outside activities, and was considered by neighbors to be an "odd duck." Her father had recently retired, and because his pension was limited, the parents were having difficulty in making ends meet. They had the added responsibility of supporting their daughter, who had been living with them for the past eight years after having been laid off from an assembly-line job she had held for about 10 years. The patient readily admitted that she preferred to be alone, but denied that this was a problem for her. She said she believed that her mother was concerned about her because of what might happen to her once her parents died. Ms. S., an only child, had graduated from high school with average grades, but had never been involved in extracurricular activities. She had never dated, and mentioned that she had a woman friend to whom she had not spoken in four years. Since moving back with her parents, she mainly stayed in her room preoccupied with reading books about astrology and casting her astrological charts. On examination, she was alert, but somewhat uncooperative. She looked older than her stated age, with moderately disheveled hair and clothing. Her speech was monotonal and deliberate. She achieved poor eye contact with the examiner. Her thinking was vague and tangential, and she expressed the belief that her fate lay in "the stars." She denied specific delusions or perceptual abnormalities. Ms. S.'s affect was constricted, except for one episode of anger when she thought the therapist was being critical.

Case Study: Schizotypal Personality Style

Belinda S. is a 37-year-old acquisitions editor for a large publisher. Her primary responsibility is to review proposals and manuscripts in science fiction and the occult to determine if her company should publish them. She finds her job fascinating and energizing, particularly since her boss has allowed her to work at home four days out of five. She has great difficulty in working a typical 9 to 5 workday as she prefers to sleep days and work at night. When reading a submitted manuscript she literally tries to put herself into the plot by imagining herself as the hero or heroine and enhances the effect by donning appropriate clothing, burning incense, and putting on suitable background music. Mark N. is her "soul mate" rather than a boyfriend. They don't actually date—he lives in another city—but spend long hours on the phone and "let their spirits commune" the rest of the time. They meet each other at various science fiction, UFO, and Star Trek conventions throughout the year.

DSM-IV Description and Criteria

In addition to having features similar to those of the schizoid personality disorder and the avoidant personality disorder, the schizotypal disorder is characterized by odd, eccentric behavior and peculiar thought content. Table 11.2 gives the DSM-IV description and criteria.

FORMULATIONS OF THE SCHIZOTYPAL PERSONALITY DISORDER

Psychodynamic Formulations

Gunderson (1988) admits that little is known about the dynamics of the schizotypal personality disorder. Gabbard (1990), among other psychoanalytically oriented writers, believes that except for a few symptoms suggestive of an attenuated form of schizophrenia, the schizoid personality and the schizotypal personality are inherently similar.

Conversely, Kellerman and Burry (1989) believe that the dynamics of the two disorders are quite different. They classify the schizoid personality disorder as an emotion-controlled character type, as with the paranoid and obsessive-compulsive personality disorders, whereas they classify the schizotypal personality disorder as an emotion-avoidant character type, along with the borderline and avoidant personality disorders.

Kellerman and Burry believe that schizotypal individuals probably experienced consistent object contact in early childhood, but that their parents failed to provide sufficient emotional closeness and warmth and were probably punitive and critical. These factors probably account for the social hypersensitivity that serves as a defense against the intense social anxiety noted in these individuals. Emotion is generally restricted, and when it is expressed, tends to be inappropriate. These individuals typically utilize a wide variety of defense mechanisms, including projection, to externalize fear and anger; a preoccupation with magical thinking and intellectualization to reduce emotional overstimulation; and hysterical denial to screen out undesirable social interactions in order to rationalize them.

Table 11.2
DSM-IV Description and Criteria for Schizotypal Personality Disorder*

301.22 Schizotypal Personality Disorder

A. A pervasive pattern of social and interpersonal deficits marked by acute discomfort with, and reduced capacity for, close relationships as well as by cognitive or perceptual distortions and eccentricities of behavior, beginning by early adulthood and present in a variety of contexts, as indicated by five (or more) of the following:

(1) ideas of reference (excluding delusions of reference)

(2) odd beliefs or magical thinking that influences behavior and is inconsistent with subcultural norms (e.g., superstitiousness, belief in clairvoyance, telepathy, or "sixth sense"; in children and adolescents, bizarre fantasies or preoccupations)

(3) unusual perceptual experiences, including bodily illusions

(4) odd thinking and speech (e.g., vague, circumstantial, metaphorical, overelaborate, or stereotyped)

(5) suspiciousness or paranoid ideation

(6) inappropriate or constricted affect

(7) behavior or appearance that is odd, eccentric, or peculiar

(8) lack of close friends or confidants other than first-degree relatives

(9) excessive social anxiety that does not diminish with familiarity and tends to be associated with paranoid fears rather than negative judgments about self

B. Does not occur exclusively during the course of Schizophrenia, a Mood Disorder With Psychotic Features, another Psychotic Disorder, or a Pervasive Developmental Disorder.

Note: If criteria are met prior to the onset of Schizophrenia, add "Premorbid," e.g., "Schizotypal Personality Disorder (Premorbid)."

*Reprinted with permission from the *Diagnostic and Statistical Manual of Mental Disorders, Fourth Edition.* Copyright 1994 American Psychiatric Association.

Biosocial Formulation

The schizotypal personality is viewed by Millon and Everly (1985) as a syndromal continuation of the schizoid and avoidant personality disorders. Thus the etiological and developmental determinants of the schizotypal disorder will be similar to those of the schizoid and avoidant disorders, but greater in intensity and chronicity. Biogenic factors in the schizotypal schizoid variant include a genetic predisposition, at least as reported in one study (Torgerson, 1984). Millon and Everly suggest that schizotypal schizoid individuals have shown a passive infantile reaction pattern that probably initiated a sequence of impoverished infantile stimulation and consequent parental indifference. Further, they point out that a dampening of the ascending reticular activity system of the limbic system may result in the autostimulation and fantasy of these individuals. Environmentally, a cold and formal family environment, combined with fragmented parental communication, probably interacts with biogenic factors to produce this personality pattern and disorder. The background of schizotypal avoidant individuals is somewhat different. Biogenically, these individuals are more likely to exhibit a "slow-to-warm-up" temperament (Thomas & Chess, 1977). They tend to be apprehensive and tense, and do not adapt quickly to new situations. Such behavior can precipitate parental tension and derogation, which further aggravates this temperament. Socially, the developmental histories of these individuals typically show parental deprecation, as well as peer and sibling humiliation, which results in interpersonal mistrust and lowered self-esteem. The continuation of these derogatory and humiliating attitudes eventually leads to self-criticism and self-deprecation.

The schizotypal personality is self-perpetuated by social isolation, overprotection, and self-insulation. Whereas social isolation and overprotectiveness have immediate benefits, in the long run they are counterproductive as they deprive these individuals of opportunities to develop social skills, in addition to fostering dependency. Furthermore, their tendency toward self-insulation serves to foster and further perpetuate the spiral of cognitive and social deterioration that typifies this disorder.

Cognitive-Behavioral Formulations

Of all the personality disorders, cognitive therapy has the least to say about schizotypal personality disorder. Nevertheless, a characteristic pattern of automatic thoughts and cognitive distortions can be discerned. Beck et al. (1990) note four types of automatic thoughts utilized by schizotypal individuals: suspicious or paranoid, ideas of reference, magical thinking, and illusions. They include such thoughts as: "Is that person watching me?" "I know they are not going to like me." "I know what she's thinking." "I feel like the devil is in him." Beck et al. indicate that oddities in cognition are the most striking feature of this disorder, and that these cognitive processes are further reflected in odd speech—circumstantial, vague, or overelaborate—as well as constricted, inappropriate affect. Typically, schizotypal individuals utilize the cognitive distortions of emotional reasoning (the belief that because they feel a negative emotion, there must be a corresponding negative external situation) and personalization (the belief that they are responsible for external situations when this is not the case).

Turkat and Maisto (1985) and Turkat (1990) describe the schizotypal personality disorder from a behavioral perspective. However, they are unable to provide a generic behavioral formulation for this disorder. Rather, Turkat (1990) notes that these patients are quite diverse in terms of behavioral presentation. This is consistent with Millon's (1981) and Millon and Everly's (1985) notion that the schizotypal personality is a decompensation of either the avoidant or schizoid personality.

Interpersonal Formulation

According to Benjamin (1993), persons diagnosed with schizotypal personality disorder probably had parents who punished them for allegedly inappropriate autonomy taking while their parents did the same. Thus the father who was rarely home might severely reprimand the child for not staying home. Essentially, such a parent modeled "mind reading," suggesting that even though he was not present, he "knew" something vitally important about the child. The adult consequence of this schizotypal modeling is that the individual imitates this pattern of "knowing" through some special means such as telepathy, mind reading, or a "sixth" sense. Parents were also likely to rely inappropriately on children to perform household duties by using threats and duress. Thus these children learned that proper behavior and obedience could avert bad outcomes. The adult consequence is the paradoxical tendency to submit to rituals that bring control. Severe abuse, often involving invasion of the children's personal boundaries, is common. Furthermore, it also is likely that strong injunctions against leaving the home for peer play or other reasons were issued by the parents. Such prohibitions interfered with the development of social feelings and skills and reinforced social isolation, as well as fantasy and autism. Finally, there is a fear of being attacked and controlled by humiliation. These individuals are prone to hostile withdrawal and self-neglect. Furthermore, they believe that they can magically influence—from a distant—circumstances and people through telepathy or ritual. Although they may be aware of their aggressive feelings, they usually constrain them.

Integrative Formulation

The following integrative formulation may be helpful in understanding how the schizotypal personality disorder is likely to develop and be maintained.

This personality disorder is described by Millon (1981) as a syndromal extension or deterioration of the schizoid or avoidant personality disorder. As such, a useful procedure is to describe the biological and temperamental features of both of these subtypes. The schizoid subtype of a schizotypal personality is characterized by a passive infantile pattern, probably resulting from low autonomic nervous system reactivity and parental indifference that led to impoverished infantile stimulation. The avoidant subtype is characterized by the fearful infantile temperamental pattern (Millon, 1981), which probably resulted from the child's high autonomic nervous system reactivity combined with parental criticalness and deprecation that was further reinforced by sibling and peer deprecation. Both subtypes of the

Table 11.3
Characteristics of Schizotypal Personality Disorder

1.	Behavioral appearance	Eccentric, erratic, bizarre; speech markedly peculiar, but not incoherent; occupationally, a dropout, drifts from job to job
2.	Interpersonal behavior	Socially isolative, peripheral relationships; intense social anxiety—apprehension or apathy; marriage—superficial relating, separation, divorce
3.	Cognitive style	"Cognitive slippage," scattered, ruminative; magical thinking, superstitious; defense is undoing (neutralize "evil" deeds, thoughts)
4.	Feeling style	Hypersensitive, hostile, and aloof
5.	Parental injunction/ environmental factors	"You're a strange bird." Cold or derogatory family environment; fragmented parental communications
6.	Biological/temperament	*Schizoid types*: passive infantile pattern—low autonomic reactivity (+) impoverished infantile stimulation/parental indifference. *Avoidance type*: fearful infantile pattern—hyperreactive temperament (+) parental/peer deprecation
7.	Self view	"I'm on a different wavelength than others." Experience of being "self-less," empty, estranged; depersonalization, dissociation
8.	World view	"Life is strange and unusual, and others have special magic intentions. Therefore, observe caution while being curious."
9.	Self and system perpetuant	Acting eccentrically (+) dependency training (+) social isolation→ increased eccentricity→ reinforcement of social isolation and differentness→ reconfirmation of schizotypal style

schizotypal personality have been noted to have impaired eye-tracking motions, which is a characteristic they share with schizophrenic individuals.

Psychologically, the schizotypals view themselves, others, the world, and life's purpose in terms of the following themes. They tend to view themselves by some variant of the theme: "I'm on a different wavelength than others." They commonly experience being self-less, that is, they experience feeling empty, estranged, and disconnected or dissociated from the rest of life. Their world view is some variant of the theme: "Life is strange and unusual, and others have special magical intentions." Thus they are likely to conclude: "Therefore, observe caution while being curious about these special magical intentions of others." The most common defense mechanism they utilize is undoing, the effort to neutralize "evil" deeds and thoughts by their eccentric beliefs and actions.

Socially, predictable patterns of parenting and environmental factors can be noted for the schizotypal personality disorder. The parenting patterns noted previously of the cold indifference of the schizoid subtype or the deprecating and derogatory parenting style and family environment of the avoidant subtype are seen here. In both cases, then, the level of functioning in the family of origin would be noted in the schizoid personality disorder or the avoidant personality disorder. Fragmented parental communications are a feature common to both subtypes of the schizotypal personality disorder. The parental injunction is likely to have been, "You're a strange bird" (Sperry & Mosak, 1993).

ASSESSMENT OF SCHIZOTYPAL PERSONALITY DISORDER

Several sources of information are useful in establishing a diagnosis and treatment plan for personality disorders. Observation, collateral information, and psychological testing are important adjuncts to the patient's self-report in the clinical interview. This section briefly describes some characteristic observations that the clinician makes and the nature of the rapport likely to develop in initial encounters with specific personality-disordered individuals. Characteristic response patterns on various objective (i.e., MMPI-2 and MCMI-II) and projective (i.e., Rorschach) tests are also described.

Interviewing patients with schizotypal personality disorders usually elicits surprising statements and peculiar ideas. Rapport is hampered as long as they feel that the clinician cannot appreciate their experiences. To the extent that the clinician is empathic and indicates understanding, they will be more willing to share their secret and autistic world. Unlike the schizoid, these individuals establish rapport easily and are usually willing to respond to all types of questions. The clinician will frequently need to ask for clarification of the impressions and constructions. Empathic listening, together with continuation techniques, is usually enough to encourage them to explain their experience. Conversely, doubting questions or confronting their views will cause them to recoil. More intelligent persons with this disorder may question whether the clinician has had experiences similar to theirs. Handling this situation is more a matter of rapport than an issue of formulating questions more effectively (Othmer & Othmer, 1989).

The Minnesota Multiphasic Personality Inventory (MMPI-2), the Millon Clinical Multiaxial Inventory (MCMI-II), and the Rorschach Psycho-diagnostic Test can be useful in diagnosing the schizotypal personality disorder, as well as the schizotypal personality style or trait.

On the MMPI-2, a 2-7-8 (Depression–Psychasthenia–Schizophrenia) code is likely for these individuals (Edell, 1987). Scales F (Frequency) and 0 (So-cial Introversion) are also likely to be elevated.

On the MCMI-II, elevations on S (Schizotypal), 2 (Avoidant), 7 (Obsessive-Compulsive), and 8A (Passive-Aggressive) can be expected (Edell, 1987; Choca et al., 1992).

On the Rorschach, these individuals have records that are more similar to those of schizophrenics and those with borderline personality disorders than to schizoid individuals (Swiercinsky, 1985).

Treatment Considerations

Included in the differential diagnosis of the schizotypal personality disor-der are three other Axis II personality disorders: schizoid personality disorder, avoidant personality disorder, and the borderline personality dis-order. The most common Axis I syndromes associated with schizotypal per-sonality disorder are the schizophrenias, particularly the disorganized, catatonic, and residual types. Other disorders noted are the anxiety disor-ders, the somataform disorders, and the dissociative disorders.

The patient with a schizotypal personality disorder finds it very diffi-cult to engage and remain in a psychotherapeutic relationship. For the ma-jority of schizotypal patients, the most realistic treatment goal is to increase their ability to function more consistently, even though on the periphery of society, rather than to have them undergo major personality restructuring.

INDIVIDUAL PSYCHOTHERAPY

Psychodynamic Psychotherapy Approaches

Individuals with schizotypal personality disorders tend to be treated in offices, clinics, and day treatment programs rather than in acute inpatient programs. They may profit from dynamically oriented psychotherapy, both expressive and supportive, depending on their level of functioning and readiness for treatment. The basis for dynamic treatment is not interpretation of conflict, but internalization of a therapeutic relationship (Stone, 1985).

Essentially, the clinician's task is to "melt" the patient's frozen internal object relations by providing a correct emotional experience. The schizotypal's style of relatedness results from inadequacies in early relationships with parental figures. As a result, these patients go through life distancing themselves from others. Therapy, therefore, must provide a new relationship for internalization (Gabbard, 1994).

Because their basic mode of functioning is nonrelational, they find the task of therapy very challenging and difficult. Not surprisingly, they respond to the challenge with silence and emotional distancing. Clinicians need to adopt a permissive, accepting attitude, and must be exceedingly patient with these individuals. It is more helpful to understand silence as a nonverbal form of relating rather than as treatment resistance. By listening with a third ear, the clinician can learn much about these patients. Through projective identification, they will evoke certain responses in the clinician that contain valuable diagnostic information regarding the patient's inner world (Gabbard, 1990). Dealing effectively with countertransference issues is critical in working with schizotypal patients. Accepting silent nonrelatedness is foreign to the clinician's psychological predisposition and training. Thus when silence is prolonged, clinicians must guard against acting out and projecting their own self and object representations onto the patient. Accepting the silence, and refraining from interpreting it, legitimizes the patient's private, noncommunicative core self. It may be the only viable technique for building a therapeutic alliance (Gabbard, 1990).

Long-Term Versus Short-Term Dynamic Therapy
Decisions about the type and frequency of dynamic therapy should be based on the patient's level of functioning and his or her motivation and readiness for treatment. More highly functioning schizotypal patients who exhibit some depressive symptoms or some capacity for empathy and emotional warmth tend to have better outcomes in dynamic psychotherapy (Stone, 1993). Similarly, patients with better ego functioning in terms of judgment, reality testing, and cognitive slippage tend to do better than those with poorer ego functioning.

Those patients who are highly motivated for exploratory psychotherapy can make dramatic gains in intense long-term treatment of two to three sessions per week over several years. On the other hand, long-term supportive psychotherapy is indicated for the majority of schizotypal patients, who present with major ego deficits and personal eccentricities. The goal of such treatment is improved adaptive functioning in day-to-day living (Stone, 1989b). Mehlum, Fris, Iron, et al. (1991) describe a long-term day treatment program for persons with schizotypal personality disorders that is based on psychodynamic principles.

Short-term dynamic therapy is indicated for crisis issues and situational difficulties related to their jobs or personal lives. It may also serve as follow-up to a previous course of long-term psychotherapy. There are few case reports of short-term dynamic individual treatment as a curative intervention.

Cognitive-Behavioral Approach

Beck et al. (1990) briefly describe the cognitive therapy approach to working with individuals with schizotypal personality disorders. Developing a collaborative working relationship is the starting point for treatment with these patients. Because they hold a number of irrational beliefs about others, the importance of the therapeutic relationship should not be underestimated. Because they desire social relationships and experience distress with social isolation, assisting them in increasing their social support network is an initial treatment goal and increasing social appropriateness is a related goal. Social skills training and the modeling of appropriate behavior and speech by the therapist are effective strategies. In combination with these behavioral strategies, the clinician should work collaboratively with the individual to identify automatic thoughts and underlying schemas about social interactions. Role playing more appropriate behavior then becomes much more meaningful.

Stone (1989b) indicates that for schizotypal patients who aspire to be able to "fit in" better and to feel less alienated, corrective training or experiences may be necessary. These may include referral to elocution lessons or a Dale Carnegie type of course, or accompanying the patient to a clothing store to assist in selecting appropriate apparel for a job interview. Stone has also found videotape feedback useful in pointing out a patient's awkwardness of gait or gestures. Turkat (1990) comments that anxiety management and modification of hypersensitivity and hypervigilance also may be necessary, depending on the case formulation.

Perhaps the most critical aspect of treatment of schizotypal individuals is helping them seek objective evidence in the environment to evaluate their thoughts, rather than relying on emotional responses. As they learn to disregard inappropriate thoughts, they are able to consider the consequences of responding emotionally or behaviorally to such thoughts, and so respond more rationally. The individual's eccentric and magical thoughts are perceived as symptoms, and predesigned coping statements—such as, "There I go again; but even though I have this thought, it doesn't mean it's true"—are practiced. In addition to guided discovery and direct disputation of maladaptive beliefs, indirect strategies, such as encouraging schizotypal patients to keep track of the predictions they make and whether the predictions were accurate, is an effective, less-threatening intervention. In addition to focusing on automatic thoughts and schemas, efforts to change the schizotypal's cognitive style are helpful. Since the communication patterns of these individuals tend to be circumstantial and idiosyncratic, collaborative experiments can be set up to modify this style. Furthermore, Beck et al. (1990) note that, provided the therapist has realistic treatment expectations, much can be accomplished, and the collaborative work can be a positive experience as these individuals are able to control portions of their inappropriate behaviors and thoughts.

Freeman et al. (1990) are not optimistic about the cognitive treatment of schizotypal individuals, indicating that behavioral interventions such as social skills training are initially useful. They point out that it is only after the actions of these individuals become more socially appropriate— that is, they begin acting more like schizoid personalities—that their automatic thoughts and cognitive distortions become amenable to cognitive methods.

Interpersonal Approach

For Benjamin (1993), psychotherapeutic interventions with persons with schizotypal personality disorders can be planned and evaluated in terms of whether they enhance collaboration, facilitate learning about maladaptive patterns and their roots, block these patterns, enhance the will to change, and effectively encourage new patterns.

The therapist facilitates collaboration by deferring to the schizotypal individual's sensitivities. For example, at the beginning of therapy, the therapist may need to be quite tolerant about canceled appointments and control over the course of sessions. If not allowed to maintain distance and control in this manner, these patients will quickly terminate. Gradually, the therapist should be able to engage them through empathic listening, accurate mirroring, and constancy. As treatment progresses, they may develop sufficient trust and insight to relinquish control by magic and ritual. Unlike parents, clinicians are not required to be caregivers. And unlike the parents of schizotypals, therapists can be consistent in mainstreaming focus and supportive attention. Such an experience is, therefore, emotionally corrective.

During the course of treatment, schizotypal individuals need to learn that the unrealistic responsibilities placed upon them when they were helpless was an abusive situation, and predisposed them to magical thinking. These early experiences led them to assume that they had inordinate power and influence. Next, they are helped to recognize when and how they distort reality. At the same time, they are taught new self-talk that can keep them grounded in the present. Later, they are helped to understand the contribution of early experiences and learnings to their unrealistic thoughts. However, for reconstructive changes to occur, these individuals must change their wish magically to protect themselves and others while maintaining their loyalty to early abusers. For example, interpreting suicidal or other fantasies in relation to underlying wishes can lead to fuller awareness, allowing the individual an opportunity for a new choice. Accurate mirroring and empathy can assist these patients to mobilize their will to recover and to visualize better ways of viewing themselves, the world, and others. Benjamin is doubtful that major changes in learning patterns will occur, however, believing that this disorder is genetically mediated.

GROUP THERAPY

Clinical reports of group therapy with schizotypal patients have been limited. Nevertheless, there is sufficient indication that these patients may profit from supportive group therapy (Stone, 1989b; Mehlum et al., 1991).

A reasonable outcome goal of group therapy is increased awareness on the part of schizotypal patients that others also harbor fantasies and self-criticisms, and that others may find them likable despite their conviction of unlikability. Group therapy may have an impact on such socially alienating tendencies as standoffishness and peculiarities of speech. An ongoing heterogeneous group may be able to tolerate such tendencies to some degree, but beyond the limits of tolerability, these behaviors may so affect either the patient or other group members that the therapeutic group process is weakened. Obviously, the selection of which schizotypal patients will benefit from being in a group is an important task for the group leaders (Stone, 1989b).

MARITAL/FAMILY THERAPY

Clinical reports of marital or family therapy with schizotypal patients have not yet appeared. In general, schizotypal patients tend to remain single. Because of either their rejection sensitivity or their insensitivity to others' feelings, they are likely to avoid committed relationships. Schizotypals who do marry tend to have problems that stem either from an insensitivity to the feelings of their partners or from an oversensitivity to the partner's behavior. Therefore, in couples therapy, the clinician's first task is to assess the degree of and balance between these two tendencies. Typically, it is easier to assist a hypersensitive partner to respond more appropriately than it is to help an insensitive partner to become more empathic (Stone, 1989b).

MEDICATION

Although there is relatively little clinical or research literature on the various psychosocial treatment modalities, there is a considerable literature on psychopharmacology for the schizotypal personality disorder. In fact, other than the borderline personality disorder, no other personality disorder has undergone as many open-trial, controlled, and placebo-controlled drug studies as the schizotypal personality disorder. The fact that this disorder lies on the schizophrenic spectrum and has some overlap with the borderline personality accounts for this interest among clinicians and researchers (Stein, 1992; Coccaro, 1993).

Several drug groups have been utilized with schizotypal patients. Anxiolytics in small doses have shown favorable responses in schizotypal patients presenting with moderate anxiety (Akiskal, 1981). Amoxapine, an antidepressant with antipsychotic properties, has been effective in improving schizophrenic-like and depressive symptoms in schizotypal patients (Jensen & Andersen, 1989). And recently, fluoxetine (Prozac) has been reported to reduce symptoms of interpersonal sensitivity, anxiety, paranoid ideation, and self-injury in both schizotypal and borderline patients (Markowitz et al., 1991).

However, the data on the effectiveness of antipsychotics for schizotypal personality disorder are most impressive. Open trials, controlled trials, and even placebo-controlled trials consistently show that low-dose antipsychotics are very beneficial for patients with moderately severe schizotypal symptoms, and have also been more effective in relieving depressive symptoms in schizotypals than have tricyclic antidepressants (Stein, 1992; Coccaro, 1993).

COMBINED AND INTEGRATED TREATMENT

Probably because of the impairing nature of this disorder, there is surprisingly little resistance to combining and tailoring treatment.

Combining medication and psychotherapy is perhaps the most common strategy. Liebowitz et al. (1986), among others, suggest beginning individual therapy and medication, where indicated, concurrently. Stone (1992) advocates beginning with medication or a behavioral intervention and adding a dimensional psychotherapy: a blending of supportive, exploratory, cognitive, and behavioral elements to match the concurrent needs and circumstances of the patient. This, of course, represents the epitome of integrated, tailored treatment.

Others have advocated social skills training as an adjunct to supportive psychotherapy (Liebowitz et al., 1986) or combining group therapy with individual dynamic psychotherapy (Gabbard, 1994). Mehlum et al. (1991) report on the combining of several treatment modalities for schizotypal and borderline personality disorders: individual psychodynamic psychotherapy, group therapy, community meetings, art therapy, awareness group therapy, and milieu therapy. This unique prospective study of a day treatment program showed that efficacy of this combined treatment approach held up an average of three years later. Major changes were noted in symptom reduction. However, social adjustments and employment were not as robust as with borderline patients.

CHAPTER 12

Personality Disorder Not Otherwise Specified (NOS)

This category of personality disorder not otherwise specified (NOS) is for disorders of personality functioning that do not meet the criteria for any specific personality disorder. An example is the presence of features of more than one specific personality disorder that do not meet the full criteria for any one personality disorder, but together cause clinically significant distress or impairment in one or more important areas of functioning (e.g., social or occupational). This category can also be used when the clinician judges that a specific personality disorder not included in this classification is appropriate. Examples include passive-aggressive personality disorder and depressive personality disorder. The passive-aggressive personality disorder, which was included in DSM-III and DSM-III-R, was relegated to Appendix B in DSM-IV because it was considered too narrowly defined and as more reflective of a symptom cluster than of a personality disorder.

This chapter describes the passive-aggressive personality disorder because it is quite commonly seen in clinical settings, and is particularly challenging for most clinicians.

PASSIVE-AGGRESSIVE PERSONALITY DISORDER

The first general use of the term "passive-aggressive personality" appeared in an armed forces technical manual in 1945, although it had been a part of the clinical literature since Kraepelin's early description in 1913. Bleuler, Schneider, Abraham, and Menninger variously described the ill-tempered, pessimistic, and discontented nature of passive aggressivity (Millon, 1993).

The diagnosis has appeared in all DSM editions. First, it was termed the passive-aggressive personality trait disturbance to describe the manner in which the disorder was expressed in military personnel during World War II. DSM-III specified passive-aggressive personality disorder as one of the disorders in the "anxious" clusters, and DSM-III-R attempted to differentiate it more clearly from the others by name criteria. Because the diagnosis was considered too situation specific and too narrowly defined, DSM-IV relegated it to an "other conditions" category. Efforts to modify it further to reflect its earlier formulation as the nail-biting character rather than the World War II formulation were unsuccessful. The proposed name change was "negative personality disorder" (Millon, 1993).

The estimated prevalence of the disorder in the general population is approximately 1 percent. Unfortunately, current data are insufficient to provide an estimate of its prevalence in clinical settings (Stone, 1993).

The remainder of this chapter describes the characteristic features of the passive-aggressive personality disorder and its related personality style. Five clinical formulations of the disorder, as well as interview and psychological assessment indicators, are highlighted. A variety of treatment approaches, modalities, and intervention stereotypes are also described.

CHARACTERISTICS OF THE PASSIVE-AGGRESSIVE PERSONALITY STYLE AND DISORDER

The passive-aggressive personality can be thought of as spanning a continuum from healthy to pathological, with the passive-aggressive personality style at the healthy end and the passive-aggressive personality disorder at the pathological end. Table 12.1 compares and contrasts the passive-aggressive personality style and disorder.

The passive-aggressive personality disorder is usually characterized by the following behavioral and interpersonal, cognitive, and affective styles.

Behaviorally, passive-aggressive persons exhibit a passive resistance to performing adequately by such means as stubbornness, forgetfulness, tardiness, deliberate inefficiency, or procrastination. Their behavior is basically oppositional and provocative in nature. They are the perennial "sour pusses." Interpersonally, they are uncooperative, and quickly dampen others' enthusiasm. They easily induce guilt in others, and Mosak (1988) has called them "injustice collectors." In relation to others, they appear to be socially ambivalent. On the one hand, they appear to be insecure, dependent, and victimized, but, on the other hand, they present themselves as provocative, independent, and oppositional.

The cognitive style of passive-aggressive individuals is characterized as conflictual. They quickly fluctuate between an assertive or defiant stance and a pleasing or reliant stance. For example, the self-talk of the passive-aggressive personality is typically: "He has no right to do that to me...I'll retaliate" (the direct aggressive and defiant stance), "but he'll really get me then" (the passive-aggressive or reliant stance) (Burns & Epstein, 1983). Passive-aggressive individuals have little awareness that their behavior is responsible for generating negative feelings and responses in others. Furthermore, their cognitive style encompasses a fault-finding type of cynicism as befitting their deeply pessimistic outlook on life.

Emotionally, passive-aggressive individuals do not show anger directly, but instead tend to sulk and become sullen. Although temper tantrums were common in them as children, temper outbursts are rarely seen in the passive-aggressive adult.

Table 12.1
Comparison of the Passive-Aggressive Style and Disorder

Personality Style	*Personality Disorder*
• Fulfill their given responsibilities.	• Resist fulfilling their given responsibilities through procrastinating, "forgetting," sulking, or being argumentative.
• Cannot be exploited, but can comfortably resist unreasonable demands.	• Protest, without justification, that unreasonable demands are being placed on them.
• Are relaxed about time, are Type B.	• Seem to work deliberately slowly or to do a bad job on tasks that they do not really want to do.
• Are cooperative with others, and comfortable with groups and family members.	• Obstruct the efforts of others and fail to do their share; are uncooperative.
• Are not overawed by authority.	• Resent useful suggestions from others concerning how they might be more productive.

The following two case examples further illustrate the differences between the passive-aggressive personality disorder (Ms. U.) and the passive-aggressive personality style (Mr. P.).

Case Study: Passive-Aggressive Personality Disorder

Ms. U. is a 37-year-old woman who was referred for counseling to a community mental health clinic by her family physician after his workup for abdominal pain proved negative. She appeared for her first therapy appointment 20 minutes late, stating that she had trouble finding a place to park. She stated that she had had abdominal pains for years and that "none of those doctors could help me." Ms. U. has had custody of her two children—now both teenagers—for the 10 years she has been divorced. She had been fired from five jobs because of chronic tardiness and forgetfulness. She smiled throughout most of the session and appeared to be compliant and cooperative, yet she indicated that she tried counseling once before but did not continue "because I didn't think it was all in my head like they tried to tell me."

Case Study: Passive-Aggressive Personality Style

Mr. P. is a 52-year-old industrial engineer who has been employed at a VA medical center ever since he graduated from college. He has been married for 30 years and has two children and three grandchildren. Over the years, Mr. P. had been offered several other jobs that would have provided higher salaries and opportunities for advancement, but he turned them all down because, he maintained, the increased pay could not offset the increased work demands, hours, and stress. Overall, he expressed satisfaction with his job, his friends at work, and the comfortable routines. Although he likes his 8:00–4:30 job well enough, he particularly enjoys evenings and weekends. In the evening, he spends long hours with his hobby of tying trout flies or playing with his grandchildren on their frequent visits. He has a mobile home, which he uses during his summer vacations and whenever else he feels like traveling and the weather permits. He has never volunteered to work overtime, is not interested in union activities, and even refused a nomination as a union representative. He said he likes his life just the way it is, and sees no need to change or modify his comfortable pattern of living.

DSM-IV Description and Criteria

Table 12.2 presents the description and research criteria as given in DSM-IV, Appendix B.

Table 12.2
DSM-IV Research Criteria for Passive-Aggressive Personality Disorder*

A. A pervasive pattern of negativistic attitudes and passive resistance to demands for adequate performance, beginning by early adulthood and present
in a variety of contexts, as indicated by four (or more) of the following:

(1) passively resists fulfilling routine social and occupational tasks

(2) complains of being misunderstood and unappreciated by others

(3) is sullen and argumentative

(4) unreasonably criticizes and scorns authority

(5) expresses envy and resentment toward those apparently more fortunate

(6) voices exaggerated and persistent complaints of personal misfortune

(7) alternates between hostile defiance and contrition

B. Does not occur exclusively during Major Depressive Episodes and is not
better accounted for by Dysthymic Disorder.

*Reprinted with permission from the *Diagnostic and Statistical Manual of Mental Disorders,
Fourth Edition.* Copyright 1994 American Psychiatric Association.

FORMULATIONS OF THE PASSIVE-AGGRESSIVE
PERSONALITY DISORDER

Psychodynamic Formulations

Compared with other disorders, the psychoanalytic literature is limited
regarding the etiology and pathogenesis of passive-aggressive behavior.
Gunderson (1983) notes that power struggles between overbearing parents
and passive-aggressive children during the anal phase of development contribute to passive aggressivity. Stricker (1983) believes that passive
aggressivity is initiated by a failure of the parenting object to meet the child's
dependency needs. This results in frustrating insecurity and anger. Because
these parents tend to be harsh or demanding, these children do not feel safe
expressing their anger directly. Rather, indirect methods are chosen, which
have the advantage of causing the parents frustration and irritation while
saving the children from having to face the consequences of their actions.
Unfortunately, such methods also have the disadvantage of creating a series of failures that undermine self-esteem and reduce the likelihood of
developing the sense of competence that comes with assuming responsibility for one's actions.

Furthermore, the mechanism of projective identification also appears
central to the development of passive aggressivity. From an object relations
perspective, self-representations associated with anger are highly unacceptable to these individuals. Thus they tend to disavow this aspect of the self

projectively and to coerce others into identifying with the projection by covertly noncompliant behavior. As projective identification operates at an unconscious level, these individuals often feel that they are completely free of anger and that others unjustly accuse them (Gabbard, 1990). Finally, Wetzler (1992) suggests that passive-aggressive individuals experience difficulty in the rapprochement subphase of separation-individuation. Like those with borderline personality disorders, they vacillate between a genuine inclination to be independent and a need for continual parental nurturance and protection.

Biosocial Formulation

Millon and Everly (1985) suggest that specific biogenic and environmental factors interact to establish the passive-aggressive pattern. They report that low stimulation thresholds within the limbic system circuitry probably give rise to affective irritability. Oldham and Morris (1990) contend that a "difficult child" temperament predisposes individuals to these disorders. Infants with this temperament frequently exhibit bad moods and dislike changes in their daily routines, especially changes in feeding and sleeping schedules. Finally, Millon (1969) suggests that passive-aggressive women may be exquisitely sensitive to hormonal changes during their menstrual cycles, which could account for their short-lived, variable moods, as in the premenstrual syndrome (PMS).

Parental inconsistency, conflictual parents, sibling rivalry, and learned vacillation are the social or environmental factors that are implicated in this disorder. Parents of passive-aggressive individuals are noted to have shifted erratically from affection to rejection and from love to hostility. Not surprisingly, their children develop a variety of pervasive and deeply ingrained conflicts, such as trust–mistrust, competence–doubt, and initiative–guilt. Constant parental conflicts, or what Millon calls "family schisms," characterize the families of passive-aggressive individuals. Typically, as children, they constantly worried about family dissolution and often attempted to play peacemaker or moderator roles. This role of switching from one point of view to another breeds ambivalence, which is a characteristic feature of passive aggressivity. Many report having been replaced in the family order by a younger sibling, a shock that can be so great that deeply rooted feelings of resentment and jealousy emerge. Upon receiving feedback that displaying such feelings is inappropriate, they learned to be sneaky, and even physically abusive toward their siblings when their parents were absent. Finally, because they repeatedly switched back and forth among a number of roles—peacemaker, martyr, victim, the misunderstood, the guilt-ridden—they quickly became familiar with the psychological benefits of learned vacillation. They were able to garner considerable attention, reassurance, and dependency, while venting their anger and frustration under the guise of social responsibility.

This disorder is perpetuated by the absence of emotional controls, the creation and anticipation of disappointment, and the reinforcement of the passive-aggressive behavior itself. Essentially, these individuals seldom learn to conceal their emotions and to develop self-control strategies, and because they have learned that good things seldom last long, they anticipate frustration, betrayal, and disappointment. This anticipation creates a self-fulfilling prophecy and further fuels their pessimistic outlook on life. Their lack of emotional control and the self-fulfilling anticipation of disappointment leads them to distrust others and to freely display their frustration and discontent.

Cognitive-Behavioral Formulations

From a cognitive therapy perspective, individuals with passive-aggressive personality disorders exhibit a characteristic pattern of schemas, assumptions, automatic thoughts, and cognitive distortions. Burns and Epstein (1983) indicate that three central assumptions or schemas are present: entitlement, or the belief that "others should meet my needs"; reciprocity, or the belief that others should be good to them because of their good behavior; and conflict phobia, or the belief that "individuals who care about each other shouldn't fight." Freeman et al. (1990) suggest that anger and justice are the underlying assumptions of this disorder. They note that passive-aggressive individuals believe that the direct expression of anger is dangerous. When this assumption is combined with assumptions about justice and fairness, chronic passive aggressiveness results: "Everyone should know the right way to treat a person, and, therefore, I should not have to ask for what I want or need." Beck et al. (1990) note that these individuals view themselves as self-sufficient but vulnerable to control and interference, while viewing the world and others as intrusive, demanding, and interfering with their freedom. Accordingly, they utilize such neurotic strategies as passive resistance, surface submissiveness, and evasion and circumvention of rules.

The automatic thoughts of passive-aggressive individuals reflect their negativity, autonomy, and desire to follow the path of least resistance. Their difficulty with being assertive stems from the belief that open conflict is terrible and will result in disapproval or rejection. Other typical automatic beliefs are: "How dare they tell me what to do," "Nobody gives me credit for all the work I do," and "Nothing ever works out for me" (Beck et al., 1990). Characteristic cognitive distortions of passive-aggressive persons include all-or-nothing thinking, mind reading, selective abstraction, and emotional reasoning (Freeman et al., 1990).

From a behavioral perspective, Turkat (1990) suggests that passive aggressivity is best formulated as a severe deficit in directly expressing emotion. He adds that some passive-aggressive individuals also have assertiveness deficits specific to a circumstance—usually involving close interpersonal relations—rather than a general deficit in assertiveness.

Interpersonal Formulation

According to Benjamin (1993), persons with passive-aggressive disorders typically have early developmental histories marked by nurturing parenting that fostered trust in the competence and constancy of caregivers. As a result, they came to expect and demand nurturance. However, this nurturance was abruptly withdrawn and replaced with unfair demands for performance. Typically, these passive-aggressive individuals were displaced as the center of attention and focus of nurturance by the birth or arrival of a younger sibling, and demands for performance were placed on them that they viewed as unfair. The adult consequence is sensitivity to power, as these individuals looked upon caregivers and authority figures as cruel, overly demanding, neglectful, and unfair. In addition, they were harshly punished for expressing anger or autonomy or for failing to submit or to perform tasks. As a consequence, they indirectly express anger and appear to comply, but actually resist demands to perform. Finally, there is a tendency to view any form of power as inconsiderate and neglectful, and to believe that all authority figures are incompetent, unfair, and cruel. They may agree to comply with demands or suggestions, but they will fail to perform. They will complain of unfair treatment, and will envy or resent others who seem to fare better. In short, they fear control in any form and constantly wish for the restitution of nurturance.

Integrative Formulation

The following integrative formulation may be helpful in understanding how the passive-aggressive personality disorder is likely to develop and be maintained.

Biologically, passive-aggressive individuals were likely to have exhibited the "difficult child" temperamental style (Thomas & Chess, 1977). Their behavior as children, adolescents, and adults was typically characterized by affective irritability. Millon and Everly (1985) suggest that low stimulation thresholds in the limbic structures of the brain probably account for this biological pattern.

Psychologically, passive aggressives' views of themselves, others, the world, and life's purposes can be articulated in terms of the following themes. They tend to view themselves by some variant of the theme: "I am competent, but not competent," and other such contradictory appraisals. They tend to view life by some variant of the theme: "Life is a big bind. It's unfair, unpredictable, and unappreciative," or "People try to push you around." And they are likely to conclude: "Therefore, vacillate, temporize, oppose, and anticipate disappointment and betrayal," or "It is better to be stubborn and get some satisfaction than to take the risk of losing everything." The Irish saying "The devil you know is better than the devil you don't know" nicely characterizes this conviction. The most likely defense mechanisms to be utilized by these individuals are displacement and projective identification.

Table 12.3
Characteristics of Passive-Aggressive Personality Disorder

1.	Behavioral appearance	Indecision, procrastination, tardiness; oppositional, forgetful, mistrustful; pessimistic; envious, "sour puss"
2.	Interpersonal behavior	Uncooperative, dampens others' enthusiasm; socially ambivalent (impulsive role shifting); insecure, dependent, victimized; guilt peddling, injustice collecting
3.	Cognitive style	Conflict—assertive (defiant) vs. pleasing (reliant); "He has no right to do X—I'll retaliate (direct anger)—but he'll really get me then" (passive anger)
4.	Feeling style	"Smiling" resistance, resentful
5.	Parental injunction/ environmental factors	"Don't count on things staying the same." Moderator/switcher role in conflicted family sibling rivalry; replaced by younger sibling
6.	Biological/temperament	"Difficult infant"; affective, irritable; hormonal/premenstrual syndrome
7.	Self view	"I'm competent, but not competent" (and other contradictory appraisals)
8.	World view	"Life is a big bind. It's unfair, unpredictable, and unappreciative. Therefore, vacillate, temporize, and anticipate disappointment and betrayal."
9.	Self and system perpetuant	Learned vacillation (+) oppositional behavior→ inconsistency and rejection→ increased ambivalence→ reinforcement of passive-aggressive style

Socially, predictable patterns of parenting and environmental factors can be noted for the passive-aggressive personality. Passive-aggressive individuals were most likely exposed to a parenting style characterized by inconsistency. Thus they might be severely disciplined for a particular infraction at one time, whereas at other times would experienced little or no discipline for the same infraction. Communication patterns were also inconsistent and contradictory. Family schisms and sibling rivalry are common features of this disorder. The passive-aggressive individual was likely to have experienced being cut off from his parents' affection by the birth of a younger sibling, resulting in an ambivalence of feelings and behavior. Sometimes he or she was chosen to play the role of moderator or peacemaker in a conflicted family. In general, contradictory thinking and behavior were reinforced in the family of origin. Learned vacillation and role switching were the family's legacy to the passive-aggressive individual.

This passive-aggressive pattern was confirmed, reinforced, and perpetuated by the following individual and systems factors: a self view of contradictory appraisals plus unpredictability and inconsistency leading to learned vacillation and role-switching behavior. The reinforcement of this ambivalent and contradictory behavior then provoked rejection by others, which led to further ambivalence and role switching, leading to further confirmation of passive-aggressive beliefs and behavior (Sperry & Mosak, 1993).

ASSESSMENT OF PASSIVE-AGGRESSIVE PERSONALITY DISORDER

Several sources of information are useful in establishing a diagnosis and treatment plan for personality disorders. Observation, collateral information, and psychological testing are important adjuncts to the patient's self-report in the clinical interview. This section briefly describes some characteristic observations that the clinician makes and the nature of the rapport likely to develop in initial encounters with specific personality-disordered individuals. Characteristic response patterns on various objective (i.e., MMPI-2 and MCMI-II) and projective (i.e., Rorschach and TAT) tests are also described.

Interviewing patients with passive-aggressive personality disorders may be quite frustrating and unrewarding. Like individuals with dependent personalities, those with passive-aggressive personalities establish and maintain rapport as long as the clinician sides and agrees with them. Challenging their views is likely to trigger their anger. They are especially sensitive to demands placed on them and react predictably, even in initial interviews. Addressing their resentment of demands must be done from their point of view; otherwise, they become guarded, monosyllabic, and hostile.

A failure to appreciate their sensitivity to demands results in a loss of rapport. Therefore, the clinician does well to explore slowly and carefully their deep aversion to standards. At the same time, the clinician must exhibit an understanding of their need for leniency, while pointing out that unfulfilled expectations cause resentment and disappointment, especially in relationships. This strategy further builds the therapeutic alliance and reduces the opportunity for pessimism, albeit it temporarily (Othmer & Othmer, 1989).

The Minnesota Multiphasic Personality Inventory (MMPI-2), the Millon Clinical Multiaxial Inventory (MCMI-II), the Rorschach Psychodiagnostic Test, and the Thematic Apperception Test (TAT) can be useful in diagnosing the passive-aggressive personality disorder, as well as the passive-aggressive personality style or trait.

On the MMPI-2, a 3-4/4-3 (Hysteria–Psychopathic Deviant) profile is common. Elevation of K (Correction) is likely, as these individuals downplay their faults and display a lack of psychological mindedness. Individuals with a 4-6/6-4 (Psychopathic Deviant–Paranoia) profile may often have difficulty controlling aggressive impulses and can have much cross-sex hostility (Meyer, 1993).

On the MCMI-II, these individuals have high elevations (above 85) on scale 8A (Passive-aggressive). Scale 6B (Sadistic) may also be elevated. While distressed, A (Anxiety) and D (Dysthymia) may be elevated, as may H (Somatoform) (Meyer, 1993).

On the Rorschach, a high percentage of Fc (Form Color) and S (Space), as well as T, FT or TF (Texture) and P (Popular), responses are likely. Odd combinations of aggressive and passive content may occur, such as guns and children, or there may be an arbitrary assignment of content or color to a space (Wagner & Wagner, 1981).

On the TAT, negativistic and avoidant themes may be prominent (Meyer, 1993).

TREATMENT APPROACHES AND INTERVENTIONS

Treatment Considerations

Included in the differential diagnosis of passive-aggressive personality disorder are other Axis II personality disorders: self-defeating personality disorder, the antisocial personality disorder, and the avoidant personality disorder. The most common Axis I syndromes associated with the passive-aggressive personality disorder are generalized anxiety disorder, dysthymia, cyclothymia, and various somatoform disorders, particularly hypochondriasis, somatization disorder, and psychophysiological disorders. In addition, factitious disorders are seen with this Axis II condition.

Treatment goals are similar to those for the dependent personality disorder—to increase the individual's ability to think and act independently and interdependently. There is a general consensus among clinicians that treatment of the patient with a passive-aggressive disorder is much less rewarding and is more frustrating than working with most of the other mild to moderate personality disorders. General treatment goals involve assertive communication and minimization of pessimism. General treatment strategies include establishing a collaborative relationship that minimizes power struggles and clarifies rules and expectations for treatment. With some patients, the suggestion is that these rules and expectations be specified in writing to stave off the kind of oppositional behavior, "forgetfulness," and argumentativeness that are frequently evoked as they test treatment limits. Methods of treatment involve both direct and indirect techniques. Insight-oriented psychotherapy has been shown to have relatively limited utility in the treatment of this disorder, as noted in the following.

INDIVIDUAL PSYCHOTHERAPIES

Many consider the passive-aggressive personality to be resistant to treatment or to be so frustrating that they choose not to work clinically with these individuals any more than they must. The major dilemma in individual psychotherapy is clearly resistance and negative transference and the clinician's negative countertransference. The negative transference is experienced as a desire to struggle to avoid giving in to the requirements of treatment or the clinician's demands. The clinician's countertransference involves annoyance, anger, and frustration. For the inexperienced clinician, the challenge is to overcome the countertransference tendency to "rescue" the patient, and to realize that the patient sees such efforts as a duplication of the early parental demands in which love was contingent on adequate performance. Regardless of the therapeutic approach or orientation, the clinician must be brave enough to let these patients fail, rather than rescue them. Individual psychotherapy then requires enormous patience, a willingness to confront the patient's opposition and pessimism, and the ability to navigate around the patient's many transference traps, criticism, and ambivalence (Liebowitz et al., 1986). These patients tend to terminate treatment prematurely, especially in the initial phase (Perry & Flannery, 1982).

Psychodynamic Approaches

Although this disorder has been artfully formulated in dynamic terms, no psychodynamic writer has addressed the issue of treatment in other than a peripheral manner. Stricker (1983) notes that the key treatment decision the clinician must make involves treatment focus and outcome goals. If there are ego-dystonic symptoms, a short-term focused and structured treatment is likely to be successful. On the other hand, ego-syntonic presentations and a focus on personality restructuring lead to long-term intensive treatment where the prognosis is guarded. Despite showing surface compliance and cooperation, these patients typically endeavor to undermine treatment.

Reich (1949) emphasized the importance of establishing a therapeutic alliance and confronting the patient's passive aggressivity in the transference, especially his or her whining and complaining. Stricker (1983) recommends the strategy of not answering the patient's numerous questions, but turning responsibility back by asking: "What do you think?" or "Why do you ask?" or "What options do you have?" This strategy is one of many used to develop self-reliance and an observing ego.

Liebowitz et al. (1986) cautioned against a supportive therapy stance, stating that giving advice invariably fails because these patients are so adroit at trivializing, criticizing, and rebutting the clinician's recommendations.

As therapy progresses and they assume a greater willingness to examine their behavior, a more searching therapeutic response can be made. As they become more willing to accept assistance, the clinician can inquire as to who in the past made decisions for them. And after the theme has been further developed, ask them how it felt to be in that position of dependency, clarifying both the angry and happy feelings. The purpose is to clarify the experience of dependency, which was frustrating and led to anger, but an anger that was inhibited and expressed passive aggressively. The relating of these early feelings to current feelings within and outside the transference can short-circuit the pathological sequence.

Countertransference issues predominate in individual treatment, particularly in dynamic treatment. In fact, Gabbard (1990) says that the diagnosis of passive-aggressive behavior may be regarded as a countertransference diagnosis. These are productive ways of handling countertransference that can undermine the therapist's view that dependency needs are doomed to frustration, that authority cannot be trusted, or that it is too dangerous to relinquish neurotic patterns. Instead, the clinician can use it to illustrate how patients undermine themselves by creating a self-fulfilling prophecy, daring others to get close to them, or defying others to supply what they desperately need and want. This, of course, requires that an adequate therapeutic alliance be formed (Stricker, 1983). Gabbard (1990) suggests asking: "I sense you're trying to make me angry with you. Do you have any idea about why you would want to do that?" Such an inquiry initially will be met with strident denial, since they cannot view themselves as completely without anger. The clinician then proceeds to identify specific aspects of their behavior that provoke anger in others. Collaboratively, the patient and clinician can search for the reasons why the patient repudiates anger and performs inadequately.

Short-Term Psychodynamic Psychotherapy
Magnavita (1993a) describes a short-term psychodynamic approach with passive-aggressive patients and compares it with cognitive and behavioral approaches. Magnavita (1993b) shows how Davanloo's intensive short-term dynamic psychotherapy has proved effective with certain passive-aggressive patients.

Cognitive-Behavioral Approach

Beck et al. (1990) provide an in-depth discussion of the cognitive therapy approach with patients with passive-aggressive personality disorders. Although these individuals are considered among the more difficult and unpleasant to work with therapeutically, Beck et al. believe that effective outcomes are possible with cognitive therapy. Several strategies are given for working with these patients. Establishing a collaborative working relationship very early in the course of treatment is absolutely essential for therapeutic progress to occur. Since these individuals defy authority figures and engage in power struggles, it is important that they realize that they are actively making choices in therapy rather than being manipulated or directed by the therapist. Collaboration can be reflected in many ways, such as the therapist's initially encouraging them to choose issues for discussion in the sessions, or jointly setting up "experiments" with them to test the accuracy of automatic thoughts or assumptions, rather than attempting to interpret or challenge these thoughts or assumptions.

A second strategy involves helping these individuals become more aware of the cognitions that influence their dysfunctional behavior and negative affects. This strategy is central to the cognitive therapy approach, and includes an analysis and restructuring of basic maladaptive schemas about passivity, autonomy, resistance, and sabotage. Maintaining consistency in treatment is another strategy. Since these patients typically blame others for their problems, it is critical that rules and limits about time, fees, telephone calls, and the like be set and followed consistently. Assisting them to examine their patterns of seeking retribution and "getting back" at others is another strategy and treatment focus. The advantages and disadvantages of this pattern should be explored and alternatives generated.

Another strategy involves facilitating and encouraging prosocial and assertive behaviors. For some, this will involve skill training. Although the basic outcome goal is for these individuals to utilize more adaptive ways of handling anger and resentment, from a cognitive therapy perspective, assertiveness training alone is insufficient. It is first necessary for passive-aggressive individuals to recognize both their passive-aggressive behavior and its consequences. Only then will it be possible collaboratively to explore other options for handling negative affects and to address the fears and expectations that block adaptive responses.

In summary, the cognitive therapy approach with passive-aggressive individuals emphasizes a collaborative working relationship, both to prevent power struggles and to provide a corrective experience, that is, the opportunity to act assertively and responsibly without fear of retribution. Besides disputing automatic thoughts and maladaptive schemas, behavioral experiments and skill training (i.e., assertion training) typically are incorporated.

Perry and Flannery (1982) proposed a behavioral approach based on assertiveness training, which is unique in that it is tailored or modified on the basis of the patient's presentation. Four different patterns of passive aggressivity are delineated: anxiety inhibited, in which a concurrent Axis I (usually dysthymia or anxiety disorder) is present; environmentally inhibited, in which the patient has an abusive spouse or employer who inhibits the patient from acting positively and assertively; resentful-vindictive, which refers to the paradiagnostic passive-aggressive patient; and the patient inhibited by existential choice, or one who has made an existential choice to remain in a difficult situation that inhibits growth (i.e., caring for a difficult, aging parent). Specific treatment guidelines are elaborated for each type.

Interpersonal Approach

For Benjamin (1993), psychotherapeutic interventions with persons with passive-aggressive personality disorders can be planned and evaluated in terms of whether they enhance collaboration, facilitate learning about maladaptive patterns and their roots, block these patterns, enhance the will to change, and effectively encourage new patterns.

Benjamin points out that the classic transference pattern of passive-aggressive individuals is to ask for help, and then to refuse it and suffer as a result. Thus developing a collaborative relationship is the major treatment challenge in working with passive-aggressive individuals. Since they expect to be injured by a negligent or cruel caregiver, they are likely to act in a way that can generate strong countertransference reactions.

As the transference unfolds, therapists must remain intact and steady in the face of the expected provocation. It is unlikely that passive-aggressive patients will be receptive to examining their maladaptive patterns until their basic agenda—proving that the therapist is abusive or incompetent—has been relinquished, at least temporarily. Benjamin provides no specific strategies for blocking maladaptive patterns or strengthening the will to relinquish these patterns, but she does say that assertiveness training can be quite useful in directly addressing their basic patterns of false compliance. She cautions, however, that this method will not succeed until the necessary preparatory work has been completed. Then, once this preparatory work has been largely accomplished, new patterns can emerge.

GROUP THERAPY

There are relatively few clinical reports and no research reports on group treatment with patients with passive-aggressive personality disorders. Opinions about the appropriateness and effectiveness of this modality vary. Gabbard (1990) believes that the group process has the potential to reduce the patient's projective disavowal of aggression. But Perry (1989) notes that these patients tend to terminate treatment prematurely, often following confrontations by other group members. However, if the clinician can encourage these passive-aggressive patients to remain in the group, their denied affects can be confronted and their expression supported. Such a group may provide these patients with their first safe interpersonal environment.

Yalom (1985) designates the "help-rejecting complainer" as one of the most difficult patients in group therapy. Passive-aggressive patients seem to fit Yalom's description of this type of patient. The effects on the group are obvious: the other members become bored, irritated, frustrated, and ultimately perplexed. Group cohesiveness tends to be undermined, as faith in the group process suffers and members experience a sense of impotence.

Peters and Grunebaum (1977) offer a treatment strategy that has been effective in both heterogeneous and homogeneous groups involving help-rejecting complainers. In a homogeneous group of such patients, this strategy is advocated to avoid the expected passive-aggressive transferences and countertransferences. Basic to these are the patients' expectations for the clinician or group leader(s) to rescue them, and their subsequent rejection of any help offered. This, of course, results in the patients' being disappointed and viewing the clinician as a persecutor. The clinician, in turn, is likely to become frustrated and angry at them. The strategy is for the clinician to avoid the role of rescuer and to sidestep any impulse to express encouragement or advice. Furthermore, the clinician outdoes negativity through irony and hyperbole. Because the clinician refuses to respond in the manner they expect, the patients are forced to adopt alternative attitudes and behaviors, which lead to a new range of choices. Hence, the strategy allows for genuine contact.

MARITAL/FAMILY THERAPY

Because family therapy focuses on the complex network of relationships that sustain the passive-aggressive personality, marital and family interventions may prove to be the most useful treatment methods currently available (Millon, 1981). Since the pattern of the passive-aggressive personality is to resist demands for adequate performance, this resistance is predictably manifest in family settings around issues of finance, sex, parenting, and communication style (Slavik, Carlson, & Sperry, 1992). This indirect expression of resistance has the effect of exerting pressure on other family members to become more demanding or to take over to accomplish a given task. But since the resistance is covert, the passive-aggressive individual comes off as being nice, soft-spoken, and perhaps even reasonable, whereas the demanding family member gets louder, more demanding, or shrewish, or even more self-righteous (Kaslow, 1983).

Passive-aggressive behavior is more "effective" than assertive communication in the marital relationship, or it would not be used so often (Burns & Epstein, 1983). Passive aggressivity "works" where more assertive behavior would be undermined, disregarded, or minimized. In addition, passive aggressivity can be an "effective" attention getter. In a marital or family system that does not recognize good or assertive behavior or support positive counteractions, any attention may be preferable to no attention (Kaslow, 1983).

Slavik, Carlson, and Sperry (1992) note that the basic issue for most couples, in which one partner is passive aggressive, is indecision or a power struggle. Accordingly, the goal of conjoint marital therapy is effective decision making or power sharing. The treatment strategy requires that there be goal alignment between the couple and the clinician, and that intervention outcomes be tailored to the particular couple. Goal alignment is essential in avoiding power struggles with the couple. The clinician is urged to accept what the couple offers as their overt treatment goal, be it sexual, financial, parental, and so on. A time-limited contract regarding treatment outcome and expectations of the clinician is essential. Usually, initial interventions are cognitive-behavioral whereas later interventions are more systemic and dynamic. If the couple is somewhat compliant, a more direct approach to increasing assertiveness and decision making is taken. With a more resistant couple, a more indirect, paradoxical approach is needed. An intermediate method is useful for most other couples. This method involves structural family therapy techniques.

Initially, treatment is aimed at specific treatment obstacles or the passive-aggressive patients, who tend to view all relational problems as caused by their partners. They believe that the world must adjust to them rather than that they should adjust to others. They justify this with beliefs regarding their "integrity," their difficulty with changing their habits, the unchangeability of their partners, their fear of being overwhelmed, and so on. As treatment proceeds, these beliefs are interpreted as pessimism regarding their efficacy in the world. Essentially then, treatment is focused on the partner's learning to accommodate both his or her issues and the other partner's issues involving decision making and power in the relationship.

MEDICATION

In discussing pharmacotherapy and personality disorders, there is general agreement that a concomitant Axis I disorder should be considered for a medication trial, or that the symptom cluster attributed to the personality disorder might be the focus of a pharmacological intervention. The exception to this rule-of-thumb seems to be the passive-aggressive personality disorder.

Although some have recommended treatment of concomitant Axis I anxiety or depressive disorders (Malinow, 1981b; Perry & Flannery, 1982; Liebowitz et al., 1986), there are little or no outcome data. Conversely, Vaillant and Perry (1985) point out that patients with passive-aggressive personality disorders can be very difficult to treat with any medication, given their propensity to oppositional behavior, noncompliance, and overdosing. With that in mind, the clinician must carefully weigh the advantages of medication use in symptom management against potential problems, especially on the effect on the therapeutic alliance.

As for medication use in passive-aggressive personality disorder per se, there is one reported clinical study involving passive-aggressive patients without a diagnosable Axis I disorder. Unfortunately, the sample size was quite small, and the medications utilized were limited to a tricyclic antidepressant and a benzodiazepine. Nevertheless, three patients showed deleterious effects from either chlorpromazine and imipramine as compared with a placebo trial (Klein, Honigfield, & Feldman, 1973). On the basis of this study, it does not appear that the use of medications is promising, but from a symptom-cluster perspective, there may be some hope. Kramer (1993) reports a case in which a patient with extreme pessimism, a core dynamic of passive aggressivity, responded very positively to fluoxetine.

COMBINED AND INTEGRATED TREATMENT APPROACHES

It seems that group therapy and marital or family therapy hold considerable potential for reversing some basic features of the passive-aggressive pattern (Millon, 1981; Peters & Grunebaum, 1977). This is not to suggest that individual psychotherapy cannot effect change, but rather that personality restructuring involves long-term intensive treatment, for which the prognosis is guarded (Stricker, 1983). Nonetheless, combining individual and group or a marital and family format might have an additive effect on treatment outcomes. Currently, the effectiveness of the adjunctive use of medication awaits research verification, particularly the value of serotonin reuptake blockers in ameliorating pessimism.

References

Abramson, R. (1993). Lorazepam for narcissistic rage. *Journal of Occupational Psychiatry, 14*, 52–55.

Adler, A. (1956). Problems in psychotherapy. *American Journal of Individual Psychology, 12*, 12–24.

Adler, A. (1964). *Problems of neurosis*. New York: Harper & Row.

Adler, G. (1985). *Borderline psychopathology and its treatment*. New York: Jason Aronson.

Adler, L. (1992). Cognitive-interpersonal treatment of avoidant personality disorder. In P. Keller & S. Heyman (Eds.), *Innovations in clinical practice: A source book*, Vol. 11. Sarasota, FL: Professional Resource Exchange.

Ahktar, S. (1990). Paranoid personality disorders: A synthesis of developmental, dynamic and descriptive features. *American Journal of Psychotherapy, 44*, 5-25.

Ahktar, S. (1987). Schizoid personality disorder: A synthesis of developmental, dynamic, and descriptive features. *American Journal of Psychotherapy, 41*, 449–518.

Akiskal, H. (1981). Subaffective disorders: Dysthymic, cyclothymic, and bipolar. II: Disorders in the borderline realm. *Psychiatric Clinics of North America, 4*, 26–46.

Alden, L. (1989). Short-term structured treatment of avoidant personality disorder. *Journal of Consulting and Clinical Psychology, 57*, 756–764.

Alden, L. (1992). Cognitive-interpersonal treatment of avoidant personality disorder. In P. Keller, S. Heyman, (Eds.), *Innovations in clinical practice: A source book*, Vol. 11. Sarasota, FL: Professional Resource Exchange.

Alexander, J., & Parsons, B. (1973). Short-term behavioral intervention with delinquent families: Impact on family process and redivisions. *Journal of Abnormal Psychology, 8*, 219–225.

Alonso, A. (1992). The shattered mirror. Treatment of a group of narcissistic patients. *Group, 16*, 210–219.

Alonso, A., & Rutan, J. (1984). The impact of object relations theory on psychodynamic group therapy. *American Journal of Psychiatry, 141*, 1376–1380.

Anderson, C. (1983). A psychoeducational program for families of patients with schizophrenia. In W. McFarlene (Ed.), *Family therapy in schizophrenia*. New York: Guilford Press.

Appel, G. (1974). An approach to the treatment of schizoid phenomena. *Psychoanalytic Review, 61*, 99–113.

Arieti, S., & Bomperad, J. (1978). *Severe and mild depression: The psychotherapeutic approach*. New York: Basic Books.

227

Azima, F. (1983). Group psychotherapy with personality disorders. In H. Kaplan & B. Sadock (Eds.), *Comprehensive group psychotherapy* (2nd ed.). Baltimore: Williams & Wilkins, pp. 262–268.

Baer, L., & Jenike, M. (1992). Personality disorders in obsessive compulsive disorder. *Psychiatric Clinics of North America, 15,* 803–812.

Balint, M. (1968). *The basic fault: Therapeutic aspects of regression.* London: Tavistock.

Balint, M., Ornstein, P., & Balint, E. (1972). *Focal psychotherapy.* London: Tavistock.

Barlow, D., & Waddell, M. (1985). Agoraphobia. In D. Barlow (Ed.), *Clinical handbook of psychological disorders: A step-by-step manual.* New York: Guilford Press.

Barnes, R. (1977). Mesoridazine (Serentil) in personality disorders: A controlled trial in adolescent patients. *Diseases of Nervous System,* April, 258–264.

Beck, A. (1967). *Cognitive therapy and the emotional disorders.* New York: International Universities Press.

Beck, A., Freeman, A., and Associates (1990). *Cognitive therapy of the personality disorders.* New York: Guilford Press.

Beck, A., Rush, A., Shaw, B., & Emery, G. (1979). *Cognitive therapy of depression.* New York: Guilford Press.

Beitman, B. (1993). Pharmacotherapy and the stages of psychotherapeutic change. In J. Oldham, M. Riba, & A. Tasman (Eds.), *American Psychiatric Press review of psychiatry,* Vol. 12. Washington, DC: American Psychiatric Press, pp. 521-540.

Bellak, L. (1993). *The T.A.T., C.A.T., and S.A.T. in clinical use* (6th ed.). Orlando, FL: Grune & Stratton.

Bellak, L., & Siegel, H. (1983). *Handbook of intensive brief and emergency psychiatry.* Larchmont, NY: CPS.

Benjamin, L. (1993). *Interpersonal diagnosis and treatment of personality disorders.* New York: Guilford Press.

Berger, P. (1987). Pharmacologic treatment for borderline personality disorder. *Bulletin of the Menninger Clinic, 51,* 277–284.

Berkowitz, D. (1985). Self-object needs and marital disharmony. *Psychoanalytic Review, 72,* 229–237.

Berkowitz, D., Shapiro, R., Sinner, M., et al. (1974). Concurrent family treatment of narcissistic disorders in adolescents. *International Journal of Psychoanalysis, 3,* 371–396.

Berman, E. (1983). The treatment of troubled couples. In L. Grinspoon (Ed.), *Psychiatric updates,* Vol. 2. Washington, DC: American Psychiatric Association.

Bernstein, D., Useda, D., & Siever, L. (1993). Paranoid personality disorder. Review of the literature and recommendations for DSM-IV. *Journal of Personality Disorders, 7,* 53–62.

Binder, J. (1979). Treatment of narcissistic problems in time-limited psychotherapy. *Psychiatric Quarterly, 51,* 257–270.

Bogdanoff, M., & Elbaum, P. (1978). Role lock: Dealing with monopolizers, isolates, helpful Hannahs, and other associated characters in group psychotherapy. *International Journal of Group Psychotherapy, 28,* 247–281.

Bonime, W. (1959). The pursuit of anxiety-laden areas in therapy of the schizoid patient. *Psychiatry, 22,* 239–244.

Buie, D., & Adler, G. (1982). The definitive treatment of the borderline personality. *International Journal of Psychoanalysis, 9,* 51–87.

Burns, D., & Epstein, N. (1983). Passive-aggressiveness: A cognitive-behavioral approach. In R. Parsons & R. Wicks (Eds.), *Passive-aggressiveness: Theory and practice.* New York: Brunner/Mazel.

Cass, D., Silvers, F., & Abrams, G. (1972). Behavior group treatment of hysterics. *Archives of General Psychiatry, 26,* 42–50.

Chessick, R. (1982). Intensive psychotherapy of a borderline patient. *Archives of General Psychiatry, 39,* 413–419.

Chessick, R. (1985). *Psychology of the self and the treatment of narcissism.* New York: Jason Aronson.

Choca, J., Shanley, L., & Denburg, E. (1992). *Interpretative guide to the Millon Clinical Multiaxial Inventory.* Washington, DC: American Psychological Association.

Chodoff, P. (1989). Histrionic personality disorder. In T. Karasu (Ed.), *Treatment of psychiatric disorders*. Washington, DC: American Psychiatric Press, pp. 2727–2735.

Clarkin, J., Marzaliali, E., & Munroe-Blum, H. (1991). Group and family treatment of borderline personality disorder. *Hospital and Community Psychiatry, 42*, 1038–1043.

Cleckley, H. (1941). *The mask of sanity*. St. Louis: Mosby.

Clinical Psychiatry News (1991). Better personality disorders therapies foreseen. September, p. 26.

Cloninger, C. (1987). A systematic method for clinical description and classification of personality variables: A proposal. *Archives of General Psychiatry, 44*, 573–588.

Cloninger, C., Svrakic, D., & Przybeck, R. (1993). A psychobiological model of temperament and character. *Archives of General Psychiatry, 50*, 975–990.

Cocarro, E. (1993). Psychopharmacologic studies in patients with personality disorders: Review and perspective. *Journal of Personality Disorders, 7*(suppl.), 181–192.

Cocarro, E., & Kavoussi, R. (1991). Biological and pharmacological aspects of borderline personality disorder. *Hospital and Community Psychiatry, 42*, 1029–1033.

Costa, P., & McCrae, R. (1990). Personality disorders and the five factor model of personality. *Journal of Personality Disorders, 4*, 362–371.

Costa, P., & McCrae, R. (1992). *The NEO personality inventory: Revised manual*. Odessa, FL: Psychological Assessment Resources.

Day, M., & Semrad, E. (1971). Group therapy with neurotics and psychotics. In H. Kaplan & B. Sadock (Eds.), *Comprehensive group psychotherapy*. Baltimore: Williams & Wilkins, pp. 566–580.

Deltito, J., & Perugi, G. (1989). A case of social phobia with avoidant personality disorder. *Comprehensive Psychiatry, 30*, 498–504.

Deltito, J., & Stam, M. (1989). Psychopharmacological treatment of avoidant personality disorder. *Comprehensive Psychiatry, 30*, 498–504.

Dick, B., & Wooff, K. (1986). An evaluation of a time-limited programme of dynamic group psychotherapy. *British Journal of Psychiatry, 148*, 159–164.

Edell, W. (1987). Relationship of borderline syndrome disorders to early schizophrenia on the MMPI. *Journal of Clinical Psychology, 43*, 163–174.

Epstein, L. (1984). An interpersonal-object relations perspective working with destructive aggression. *Contemporary Psychoanalysis, 20*, 651–662.

Evans, K., & Sullivan, J. (1990). *Dual diagnosis. Counseling the mentally ill substance abuser*. New York: Guilford Press.

Everett, S., Halperin, S., Volgy, S., & Wissler, A. (1989). *Treating the borderline family: A systematic approach*. Boston: Allyn & Bacon.

Ewenbach, B., Winstead, B., & Derlega, V. (1989). Sex differences in diagnosis and treatment recommendations for antisocial personality and somatization disorders. *Journal of Social and Clinical Psychology, 8*, 238–255.

Exner, J. (1986). *The Rorschach: A comprehensive system* (2nd ed.). New York: Wiley.

Fairburn, W. (1954). *An object-relations theory of the personality*. New York: Basic Books.

Fay, A., & Lazarus, A. (1993). Cognitive-behavior group therapy. In A. Alonso & H. Swiller (Eds.), *Group therapy in clinical practice*. Washington, DC: American Psychiatric Press.

Feldman, L. (1982). Dysfunctional marital conflict: An integrative interpersonal intrapsychic model. *Journal of Marital and Family Therapy, 8*, 417–428.

Fenichel, O. (1945). *The psychoanalytic theory of the neurosis*. New York: Norton.

Fernbach, B., Winstead, B. & Derlega, V. (1989). Sex differences in diagnosis and treatment recommendations for antisocial personality and somatization disorders. *Journal of Social and Clinical Psychology, 8*: 238–255.

Fieve, R. (1994). *Prozac*. New York: Avon Books.

Finn, B., & Shakir, S. (1990). Intensive group psychotherapy of borderline patients. *Group, 14*, 99–110.

Flegenheimer, W. (1982). *Techniques of brief psychotherapy*. New York: Jason Aronson.

Fraiberg, S. (1969). Libidinal object constancy and mental representation. *Psychoanalytic Study of the Child, 24*, 9–47.

Frances, A., & Clarkin, J. (1981). Differential therapeutics: A guide to treatment selection. *Hospital and Community Psychiatry, 32*, 537–546.

Frances, A., Clarkin, J., & Perry, S. (1984). *Differential therapeutics in psychiatry: The art and science of treatment selection*. New York: Brunner/Mazel.

Freeman, A., Pretzer, J., Fleming, B., & Simon, K. (1990). *Clinical application of cognitive therapy*. New York: Plenum.

Freud, S. (1914/1976). On narcissism: An introduction. *Complete psychological works, standard edition*, Vol. 14. London: Hogarth Press, pp. 69–102.

Frosch, J. (1983). *The psychotic process*. New York: International Universities Press.

Gabbard, G. (1989). On "doing nothing" in the psychoanalytic treatment of the refractory borderline patient. *International Journal of Psychoanalysis, 70*, 527–534.

Gabbard, G. (1990). *Psychodynamic psychiatry in clinical practice*. Washington, DC: American Psychiatric Press.

Gabbard, G. (1994). *Psychodynamic psychiatry in clinical practice: The DSM-IV edition*. Washington, DC: American Psychiatric Press.

Gertsley, L., McLellan, T., Atterman, A., et al. (1989). Ability to form an alliance with the therapist: A possible marker of progress for patients with antisocial personality disorder. *American Journal of Psychiatry, 146*, 508–512.

Glantz. K., & Goisman, R. (1990). Relaxation and merging in the treatment of personality disorders. *American Journal of Psychotherapy, 44*, 405–413.

Glueck, S., & Glueck, E. (1950). *Unraveling juvenile delinquency*. Cambridge, MA: Harvard University Press.

Goldberg, A. (1973). Psychotherapy of narcissistic injuries. *Archives of General Psychiatry, 28*, 722–726.

Goldberg, A. (1989). Self psychology and the narcissistic personality disorders. *Psychiatric Clinics of North America, 12*, 731–739.

Graham, J. (1990). *MMPI-2: Assessing personality and psychopathy*. New York: Oxford.

Greist, J., & Jefferson, J. (1992). *Panic disorder and agoraphobia: A guide*. Madison, WI: Anxiety Disorders Center and Information Centers.

Grotjahn, M. (1984). The narcissistic person in analytic group psychotherapy. *International Journal of Group Psychotherapy, 30*, 299–318.

Guerney, B. (1977). *Relationship enhancement: Skill-training programs for therapy, problem prevention, and enrichment*. San Francisco: Jossey-Bass.

Guidano, V., & Liotti, G. (1983). *Cognitive processes and emotional disorders*. New York: Guilford Press.

Gunderson, J. (1980). Personality disorders. In A. Nichols (Ed.), *The new Harvard guide to psychiatry*. Cambridge, MA: Harvard University Press, pp. 337–357.

Gunderson, J. (1983). DSM-III diagnosis of personality disorders. In J. Frosch (Ed.), *Current perspectives on personality disorders*. Washington, DC: American Psychiatric Press.

Gunderson, J. (1986). Pharmacotherapy for patients with borderline personality disorders. *Archives of General Psychiatry, 43*, 698–700.

Gunderson, J. (1989). Borderline personality disorder. In T. Karasu (Ed.), *Treatments of psychiatric disorders*. Washington, DC: American Psychiatric Press, pp. 2749–2758.

Gunderson, J., Ronningstam, E., & Smith, L. (1991). Narcissistic personality disorders: A review of data on DSM-III-R descriptions. *Journal of Personality Disorders, 5*, 167–177.

Gurman, A., & Kniskern, D. (1981). Family therapy outcomes research: Known and unknown. In A. Gurman & D. Kniskern (Eds.), *Handbook of family therapy*. New York: Brunner/Mazel.

Haley, J. (1978). *Problem solving therapy*. San Francisco: Jossey-Bass.

Haley, J., & Hoffman, L. (1967). *Techniques of family therapy*. New York: Basic Books.

Halleck, S. (1978). *The treatment of emotional disorders*. New York: Jason Aronson.

Handler, L. (1989). Utilization approaches and psychodynamic psychotherapy in a case of hospital phobia: An integrated approach. *American Journal of Clinical Hypnosis, 31*, 257–263.

Harbir, H. (1981). Family therapy with personality disorders. In J. Lion (Ed.), *Personality disorders: Diagnosis and management* (2nd ed.). Baltimore: Williams & Wilkins.

Harwood, I. (1992). Advances in group psychotherapy and self psychology: An interobjective approach with narcissistic and borderline patients. *Group, 16*, 220–232.

Havens, L. (1976). Discussion: How long the Tower of Babel? *Proceedings of American Psychopathological Association, 64,* 62–73.

Heard, H., & Linehan, M. (1994). Dialectical behavior therapy: An integrative approach to the treatment of the borderline personality disorder. *Journal of Psychotherapy Integration, 4,* 55–82.

Heimberg, R., Holt, C., Schneier, F., et al. (1943). The issue of subtypes in the diagnosis of social phobia. *Journal of Anxiety Disorders, 7,* 249–269.

Hend, S., Baker, J., & Williamson, D. (1991). Family environment characteristics and dependent personality disorder. *Journal of Personality Disorders, 5,* 256–263.

Hill, D. (1970). Outpatient management of passive dependent women. *Hospital and Community Psychiatry, 21,* 402–405.

Hirschfield, R., Shea, M., & Weise, R. (1991). Dependent personality disorder: Perspective for DSM-IV. *Journal of Personality Disorders, 5,* 135–149.

Horowitz, L. (1980). Group psychotherapy for borderline and narcissistic patients. *Bulletin of the Menninger Clinic, 4,* 181–200.

Horowitz, L. (1977). Group psychotherapy of the borderline. In P. Harticollis (Ed.), *Borderline personality disorder.* New York: International Universities Press, pp. 399–422.

Horowitz, M. (1988). *Introduction to psychodynamics: A new synthesis.* New York: Basic Books.

Horowitz, M., Marmar, C., Krupnick, J., et al. (1984). *Personality styles and brief psychotherapy.* New York: Basic Books.

Hulse, W. (1958). Psychotherapy with ambulatory schizophrenic patients in mixed analytic groups. *Archives of Neurology and Psychiatry, 79,* 681–687.

Jenike, M. (1990). Approaches to the patient with treatment refractory obsessive-compulsive disorder. *Journal of Clinical Psychiatry, 51*(2, suppl.), 15–21.

Jenike, M. (1991). Obsessive-compulsive disorder. In B. Beitman & G. Klerman (Eds.), *Integrating pharmacotherapy and psychotherapy.* Washington, DC: American Psychiatric Press, pp. 183–210.

Jenike, M., Baer, L., & Minichiello, W. (1990). *Obsessive-compulsive disorders: Theory and management* (2nd ed.). Chicago: Yearbook.

Jensen, H., & Andersen, J. (1989). An open, noncomparative study of amoxapine in borderline patients. *Acta Psychiatrica Scandinavica, 79,* 89–93.

Jones, S. (1987). Family therapy with borderline and narcissistic patients. *Bulletin of the Menninger Clinic, 51,* 285–295.

Kagan, J., Reznick, J., & Snidman, N. (1988). Biological basis of childhood shyness. *Science, 240,* 161–171.

Kalus, O., Bernstein, D., & Siever, L. (1993). Schizoid personality disorder: A review of current status and implications for DSM-IV. *Journal of Personality Disorders, 7,* 43–52.

Kantor, M. (1992). *Diagnosis and treatment of the personality disorders.* St. Louis: Ishiyaku EuroAmerica.

Karasu, T. (1990). *Psychotherapy for depression.* Northvale, NJ: Jason Aronson.

Kaslow, F. (1983). Passive-aggressiveness: An intrapsychic, interpersonal and transactional dynamic in the family system. In R. Parsons & R. Wicks (Eds.), *Passive-aggressiveness: Theory and practice.* New York: Brunner/Mazel.

Kavoussi, R., Liu, J., & Coccaro, E. (1994). An open trial of sertraline in personality disordered patients with impulsive aggression. *Journal of Clinical Psychiatry, 55,* 137–141.

Kellerman, H., & Burry, A. (1989). *Psychopathology and the differential diagnosis.* Vol. II: *Diagnostic primer.* New York: Columbia University Press.

Kellner, R. (1978). Drug treatment of personality disorders and delinquents. In W. Reid (Ed.), *The psychopath: A comprehensive study of antisocial disorders and behaviors.* New York: Brunner/Mazel.

Kellner, R. (1986). Personality disorders. *Psychotherapy and Psychosomatics, 46,* 58–66.

Kernberg, O. (1975). *Borderline conditions and pathological narcissism.* New York: Jason Aronson.

Kernberg, O. (1984). *Severe personality disorders: Psychotherapeutic strategies.* New Haven, CT: Yale University Press.

Khan, M. (1975). Grudge and the hysteric. *International Journal of Psychoanalysis and Psychotherapy, 44,* 349–357.

Klein, D. (1975). Psychopharmacology and the borderline patient. In J. Mack (Ed.), *Borderline states in psychiatry*. New York: Grune & Stratton.

Klein, D., Honigfield, G., & Feldman, S. (1973). Prediction of drug effect in personality disorders. *Journal of Nervous and Mental Disease, 156,* 183–198.

Klein, R. (1989a). Diagnosis and treatment of the lower-level borderline patient. In J. Masterson & R. Klein (Eds.), *Psychotherapy of disorders of the self*. New York: Brunner/Mazel.

Klein, R. (1989b). Shorter-term psychotherapy of the personality disorders. In J. Masterson & R. Klein (Eds.), *Psychotherapy of disorders of the self*. New York: Brunner/Mazel, pp. 90–109.

Klein, R. (1989c). Pharmacotherapy of the borderline personality disorder. In J. Masterson & R. Klein (Eds.), *Psychotherapy of disorders of the self*. New York: Brunner/Mazel, pp. 365–394.

Klerman, G., & Weissman, M. (1984). *Interpersonal psychotherapy for depression*. New York: Basic Books.

Klerman, G., & Weissman, M. (Eds.). (1993). *New applications of interpersonal psychotherapy*. Washington, DC: American Psychiatric Press.

Koenigsberg, H. (1993). Combining psychotherapy and pharmacotherapy in the treatment of borderline patients. In J. Oldham, M. Riba, & A. Tasman (Eds.), *American Psychiatric Press review of psychiatry*, Vol. 12. Washington, DC: American Psychiatric Press, pp. 541–564.

Kohut, H. (1971). *The analysis of the self*. New York: International Universities Press.

Kohut, H. (1977). *The restoration of the self*. New York: International Universities Press.

Kramer, P. (1993). *Listening to Prozac*. New York: Viking.

Lachar, D. (1974). *The MMPI: Clinical assessment and automated interpretation*. Los Angeles: Western Psychological Services.

Lachkar, J. (1986). Narcissistic/borderline couples. Implications for medication. *Conciliation Courts Review, 24,* 31–38.

Lachkar, J. (1992). *The narcissistic/borderline couple: A psychoanalytic perspective on marital treatment*. New York: Brunner/Mazel.

Lazarus, A. (1981). *The practice of multimodal therapy*. New York: McGraw-Hill.

Lazarus, L. (1982). Brief psychotherapy of narcissistic disturbances. *Psychotherapy: Theory, Research, and Practice, 19,* 228–236.

Lazarus, A. (Ed.). (1985). *Casebook of multimodal therapy*. New York: Guilford Press.

Leszcz. M. (1989). Group psychotherapy of the characterologically difficult patient. *International Journal of Group Psychotherapy, 39,* 311–335.

Lewinsohn, P. (1975). Engagement in pleasant activities and depression level. *Journal of Abnormal Psychology, 84,* 729–731.

Lewinsohn, P., Antonuccio, D., Steinmetz, J., et al. (1984). *The coping with depression course: A psychoeducational intervention for unipolar depression*. Eugene, OR: Castalia Publishing.

Liebowitz, M., & Klein, D. (1981). Interrelationship of hysteroid dysphoria and borderline personality disorder. *Psychiatric Clinics of North America, 4,* 67–87.

Liebowitz, M., Schneier, F., Hollander, E., et al. (1991). Treatment of social phobia with drugs other than benzodiazepines. *Journal of Clinical Psychiatry, 52* (11, suppl.), 10–15.

Liebowitz, M., Stone, M., & Turkat, I. (1986). Treatment of personality disorders. In A. Francis & R. Hales (Eds.), *Psychiatric update, American Psychiatric Association annual review*, Vol. 5. Washington, DC: American Psychiatric Press, pp. 356–393.

Linehan, M. (1983). *Dialectical behavior therapy for treatment of parasuicidal women: Treatment manual*. Seattle: University of Washington.

Linehan, M. (1987). Dialectical behavior therapy for borderline personality disorder: Therapy and method. *Bulletin of the Menninger Clinic, 51,* 261–276.

Linehan, M. (1993). *Cognitive-behavioral treatment for borderline personality disorder*. New York: Guilford Press.

Linehan, M., Armstrong, H., Suarez, A., et al. (1991). Cognitive-behavioral treatment of chronically parasuicidal borderline patients. *Archives of General Psychiatry, 48,* 1060–1064.

Luborsky, L. (1984). *Principles of psychoanalytic psychotherapy: A manual for supportive expressive treatment*. New York: Basic Books.

Mackinnon, R., & Michels, R. (1971). *The psychiatric interview in clinical practice*. Philadelphia: Saunders.

Magnavita, J. (1993a). The treatment of passive-aggressive personality disorder: A review of current approaches: I. *International Journal of Short-Term Psychotherapy, 8,* 29–41.

Magnavita, J. (1993b). The treatment of passive-aggressive personality disorder: Intensive short-term dynamic psychotherapy: II. Trial therapy. *International Journal of Short-Term Psychotherapy, 8,* 93–106.

Malan, D. (1976). *The frontier of brief psychotherapy: An example of the convergence of research and clinical practice.* New York: Plenum.

Malinow, K. (1981a). Dependent personality. In J. Lion (Ed.), *Personality disorders: Diagnosis and management* (2nd ed.). Baltimore: Williams & Wilkins.

Malinow, K. (1981b). Passive-aggressive personality. In J. Lion (Ed.), *Personality disorders: Diagnosis and management* (2nd ed.). Baltimore: Williams & Wilkins.

Mann, J. (1973). *Time-limited psychotherapy.* Cambridge, MA: Harvard University Press.

Mann, J. (1984). Time-limited psychotherapy. In L. Grinspoon (Ed.), *Psychiatry update,* Vol. 3. Washington, DC: American Psychiatric Association.

Manschreck, T. (1992). Delusional disorders: Clinical concepts and diagnostic strategies. *Psychiatric Annals, 22,* 241–251.

Markowitz, P., Calabrese, J., Schulz, S., & Meltzer, H. (1991). Fluoxetine in the treatment of borderline and schizotypal personality disorders. *American Journal of Psychiatry, 148,* 1064–1067.

Marmar, C., & Freeman, M. (1988). Brief dynamic psychotherapy of post-traumatic stress disorders: Management of narcissistic regression. *Journal of Traumatic Stress, 1,* 323–337.

Masterson, J. (1976). *Psychotherapy of the borderline adult: A developmental approach.* New York: Brunner/Mazel.

Masterson, J. (1981). *The narcissistic and borderline disorders.* New York: Brunner/Mazel.

Masterson, J., & Klein, R. (Eds.). (1990). *Psychotherapy of the disorders of the self.* New York: Brunner/Mazel.

Masterson, J., & Orcutt, C. (1989). Marital co-therapy of a narcissistic couple. In J. Masterson & R. Klein (Eds.), *Psychotherapy of the disorders of the self.* New York: Brunner/Mazel.

Mavissakalian, M. (1993). Combined behavioral and pharmacological treatment of anxiety disorders. In J. Oldham, M. Riba, & A. Tasman (Eds.), *American Psychiatric Press review of psychiatry,* Vol. 12. Washington, DC: American Psychiatric Press, pp. 541–564.

McCormack, C. (1989). The borderline/schizoid marriage: The holding environment as an essential treatment construct. *Journal of Marital and Family Therapy, 15,* 299–309.

Megargee, E., & Bohn, M. (1979). *Classifying criminal offenders.* Beverly Hills, CA: Sage.

Mehlum, L., Fris, S., Iron, T., et al. (1991). Personality disorders 2-5 years after treatment: A prospective follow-up study. *Acta Psychiatrica Scandinavica, 84,* 72–77.

Meichenbaum, D. (1977). *Cognitive-behavioral modification: An integrated approach.* New York: Plenum.

Meissner, W. (1978). *The paranoid process.* New York: Jason Aronson.

Meissner, W. (1986). *Psychotherapy and the paranoid process.* Northvale, NJ: Jason Aronson.

Meissner, W. (1988). *Treatment of patients in the borderline spectrum.* New York: Jason Aronson.

Meissner, W. (1989). Paranoid personality disorder. In T. Karasu (Ed.), *Treatments of psychiatric disorders.* Washington, DC: American Psychiatric Press, pp. 2705–2711.

Meloy, J. (1988). *The psychopathic mind: Origins, dynamics, and treatment.* Northvale, NJ: Jason Aronson.

Meyer, R. (1993). *The clinician's handbook: Integrated diagnostics, assessment, and intervention in adult and adolescent psychotherapy.* Boston: Allyn & Bacon.

Millon, T. (1969). *Modern psychopathology: A biosocial approach to maladaptive learning and functioning.* Philadelphia: Saunders.

Millon, T. (1981). *Disorders of personality. DSM-III, Axis II.* New York: Wiley.

Millon, T. (1985). "The MCMI provides a good assessment of DSM-III disorders: The MCMI-II will prove even better." *Journal of Personality Assessment, 49,* 379–391.

Millon, T. (1990). *Toward a new personology: An evolutional model.* New York: Wiley.

Millon, T. (1993). Negativistic (passive-aggressive) personality disorder: Special feature. DSM-IV reviews of the personality disorders: III. *Journal of Personality Disorders, 7,* 78–85.

Millon, T., & Everly, G. (1985). *Personality and its disorders: A biosocial learning approach.* New York: Wiley.

Minuchin, S. (1974). *Families and family therapy*. Cambridge, MA: Harvard University Press.

Minuchin, S., Montalva, B., Guerney, B., Rosman, B. & Schumer, F. (1967). *Families of the slums*. New York: Basic Books.

Montgomery, J. (1971). Treatment management of passive-dependent behavior. *International Journal of Social Psychiatry, 17,* 311–319.

Mosak, H. (1988). "Personality disorders" in course syllabus outline. *Psychodynamics of psychopathology I and II*. Chicago: Alfred Adler Institute.

Munich, R. (1986). Transitory symptom formation in the analysis of an obsessional character. *Psychoanalytic Study of the Child, 41,* 515–535.

Munoz, R., & Ying, Y. (1993). *The prevention of depression: Research and practice*. Baltimore: Johns Hopkins University Press.

Munro, A. (1992). Psychiatric disorders characterized by delusions: Treatment in relation to specific types. *Psychiatric Annals, 22,* 232–240.

Nachmani, G. (1984). Hesitation, perplexity, and annoyance at opportunity. *Contemporary Psychoanalysis, 20,* 448, 457.

Nehls, N. (1991). Borderline personality disorder and group therapy. *Archives of Psychiatric Nursing, 5,* 137–146.

Nehls, N., & Diamond, R. (1993). Developing a systems approach to caring for persons with borderline personality disorder. *Community Mental Health Journal, 29,* 161–172.

Nemiah, J. (1980). Obsessive compulsive neurosis. In A. Freedman, H. Kaplan, & B. Sadock (Eds.), *A comprehensive textbook of psychiatry*. Baltimore: Williams & Wilkins.

Oldham, J. (1988). Brief treatment of narcissistic personality disorder. *Journal of Personality Disorders, 2,* 88–90.

Oldham, J., & Morris, L. (1990). *The personality self-portrait*. New York: Bantam.

O'Leary, K., Turner, E., Gardner, D., et al. (1991). Homogeneous group therapy for borderline personality disorder. *Group, 15,* 56–64.

Othmer, E. Othmer, S. (1989). *The clinical interview using DSM-III-R*. Washington, DC: American Psychiatric Press.

Parsons, B., & Alexander, J. (1973). Short-term family interventions: A therapy outcome study. *Journal of Abnormal Psychology, 8,* 219–225.

Perry, C., & Flannery, R. (1982). Passive-aggressive personality disorder: Treatment implications of a clinical typology. *Journal of Nervous and Mental Disease, 170,* 164–173.

Perry, J. (1989). Passive-aggressive personality disorder. In T. Karasu (Ed.), *Treatments of psychiatric disorders*. Vol. I. Washington, DC: American Psychiatric Press, pp. 2783-2789.

Perry, J., Frances, A., & Clarkin, J. (1990). *A DSM-III-R casebook of treatment selection*. New York: Brunner/Mazel.

Peters, C., & Grunebaum, H. (1977). It could be worse: Effective group psychotherapy with the help-rejecting complainer. *International Journal of Group Psychotherapy, 27,* 471–480.

Pfohl, B. (1991). Histrionic personality disorder: A review of available data and recommendations for DSM-IV. *Journal of Personality Disorders, 5,* 150–166.

Pfohl, B., & Blum, N. (1991). Obsessive-compulsive personality disorder: A review of available data and recommendations for DSM-IV. *Journal of Personality Disorders, 5,* 363–375.

Pies, R. (1992). The psychopharmacology of personality disorders. *Psychiatric Times*, February, 23–24.

Pines, M. (1975). Group psychotherapy with difficult patients. In L. Wolberg & M. Aronson (Eds.), *Group therapy 1975: An overview*. New York: Stratton Intercontinental Medical Books.

Pretzer, J. (1988). Paranoid personality disorder: A cognitive view. *International Cognitive Therapy Newsletter, 4,* 10–12.

Quality Assurance Project (1991). Treatment outlines for borderline, narcissistic and histrionic personality disorder. *Australia New Zealand Journal of Psychiatry, 25,* 392–403.

Ratey, J., Morrill, R., & Oxenburg, G. (1983). Use of propranolol for provoked and unprovoked episodes of rage. *American Journal of Psychiatry, 140,* 1356–1357.

Regier, D., Boyd, J., Burke, J., et al. (1988). One-month prevalence in mental disorders in the United States. *Archives of General Psychiatry, 45,* 977–986.

Reich, J. (1988). DSM-III personality disorders and the outcome of treated panic disorder. *American Journal of Psychiatry, 145,* 1149–1152.

Reich, W. (1949). *Character analysis* (3rd ed.). New York: Farrar, Straus, Giroux.

Reid, W. (1989). *The treatment of psychiatric disorders. Revised for the DSM-III-R*. New York: Brunner/Mazel.

Reid, W., & Burke, W. (1989). Antisocial personality disorder. In T. Karasu (Ed.), *Treatments of psychiatric disorders*. Washington, DC: American Psychiatric Press.

Rennenberg, B., Goldstein, A., Phillips, D., et al. (1990). Intensive behavioral group treatment of avoidant personality disorder. *Behavior Therapy, 21*, 363–377.

Reyntjens, A. (1972). A series of multicentric pilot trials with pimozide in psychiatric practice. I: Pimozide in the treatment of personality disorders. *Acta Psychiatria Belgeimum, 72*, 653–661.

Rinsley, D. (1982). *Borderline and other self disorders*. New York: Jason Aronson.

Rush, A., & Hollon, S. (1991). Depression. In B. Beitman & G. Klerman (Eds.), *Integrating pharmacotherapy and psychotherapy*. Washington, DC: American Psychiatric Press, pp. 121–142.

Sadoff, R., & Collins, D. (1968). Passive dependency in stutterers. *American Journal of Psychiatry, 124*, 1126–1127.

Salkovskis, P., & Kirk, J. (1989). Obsessional disorders. In K. Hawton, P. Salkovskis, J. Kirk, & D. Clark (Eds.), *Cognitive behavior therapy for psychiatric problems*. Oxford: Oxford University Press, pp. 129-168.

Salzman, L. (1980). *Treatment of the obsessive personality*. New York: Jason Aronson.

Salzman, L. (1989). Compulsive personality disorder. In T. Karasu (Ed.), *Treatment of psychiatric disorders*. Washington, DC: American Psychiatric Press, pp. 2771–2782.

Satterfield, J., & Contwell, D. (1975). Psychopharmacology in the prevention of antisocial and delinquent behavior. *International Journal of Mental Health, 4*, 227–337.

Schane, M., & Kovel, V. (1988). Family therapy in severe borderline personality disorder. *International Journal of Family Psychiatry, 9*, 241–258.

Shafer, R. (1954). *Psychoanalytic interpretations in Rorschach testing*. New York: Grune & Stratton.

Shapiro, D. (1965). *Neurotic styles*. New York: Basic Books.

Shapiro, E. (1982). The holding environment and family therapy for acting out adolescents. *International Journal of Psychoanalysis, 9*, 209–226.

Sheard, M. (1976). The effects of lithium on impulsive aggressive behavior in man. *American Journal of Psychiatry, 133*, 1409–1413.

Sheidlinger, S., & Porter, K. (1980). Group therapy combined with individual psychotherapy. In T. Karasu & L. Bellack (Eds.), *Specialized techniques in individual psychotherapy*. New York: Brunner/Mazel.

Sheldon, W., & Stevens, S. (1942). *The varieties of temperament: A psychology of constitutional differences*. New York: Harper.

Shulman, B. (1982). An Adlerian interpretation of the borderline personality. *Modern Psychoanalysis, 7*, 137–153.

Siever, L. (1993). The frontiers of psychopharmacology. *Psychology Today, 27*(1), 40–44, 70–72.

Siever, L., Bernstein, D., & Silverman, J. (1991). Schizotypal personality disorder: A review of its current status. *Journal of Personality Disorders, 5*, 178–193.

Siever, L., & Davis, K. (1991). A psychological perspective on the personality disorders. *American Journal of Psychiatry, 148*, 37–48.

Sifneos, P. (1972). *Short-term psychotherapy and emotional crisis*. Cambridge, MA: Harvard University Press.

Sifneos, P. (1984). The current status of short-term dynamic psychotherapy and its future: An overview. *American Journal of Psychotherapy, 38*, 472–487.

Slavik, S., Carlson, J., & Sperry, L. (1992). Adlerian marital therapy with the passive-aggressive partner. *American Journal of Family Therapy, 20*, 25–35.

Slavik, S., Sperry, L., & Carlson, J. (1992). The schizoid personality disorder: A review and an Adlerian view and treatment. *Individual Psychotherapy, 7*, 137–154.

Slavson, S. (1964). *A textbook in analytic group psychotherapy*. New York: International Universities Press.

Slavson, S. (1939). *Dynamics of group psychotherapy*. New York: Jason Aronson.

Snyder, M. (1994). Couple therapy with narcissistically vulnerable clients. Using the relationship enhancement model. *Family Journal: Counseling and Therapy for Couples and Families,* 2, 27–35.

Solomon, M. (1989). *Narcissism and intimacy: Love and marriage in an age of confusion.* New York: Plenum.

Sperry, L. (1990). Personality disorders: Biopsychosocial descriptions and dynamics. *Individual Psychology,* 46, 193–202.

Sperry, L. (1991a). The neurotic personalities of our time: Part I: The borderline personality. *NASAP Newsletter,* 24(6), 3–5.

Sperry, L. (1991b). The neurotic personalities of our time: Part II: The narcissistic personality. *NASAP Newsletter,* 24(9), 3–6.

Sperry, L., Gudeman, J., Blackwell, B., & Faulkner, L. (1992). *Psychiatric case formulations.* Washington, DC: American Psychiatric Press.

Sperry, L., & Mosak, H. (1993). Personality disorders. In L. Sperry & J. Carlson (Eds.), *Psychopathology and psychotherapy: From diagnosis to treatment.* Muncie, IN: Accelerated Development.

Spotnitz, H. (1975). The borderline schizophrenic in group psychotherapy. *International Journal of Group Psychotherapy,* 7, 155–174.

Stein, G. (1992). Drug treatment of the personality disorders. *British Journal of Psychiatry,* 161, 167–184.

Stone, M. (1985). Schizotypal personality: Psychotherapeutic aspects. *Schizophrenia Bulletin,* 11, 576–589.

Stone, M. (1989a). Schizoid personality disorder. In T. Karasu (Ed.), *Treatments of psychiatric disorders.* Washington, DC: American Psychiatric Press, pp. 2712–2718.

Stone, M. (1989b). Schizotypal personality disorder. In T. Karasu (Ed.), *Treatments of psychiatric disorders.* Washington, DC: American Psychiatric Press, pp. 2719–2726.

Stone, M. (1992). Treatment of severe personality disorders. In A. Tasman & M. Riba (Eds.), *American Psychiatric Press review of psychiatry,* Vol. II. Washington, DC: American Psychiatric Press, pp. 98–115.

Stone, M. (1993). *Abnormalities of personality: Within and beyond the realm of treatment.* New York: Norton.

Stone, M., & Weissman, R. (1984). Group therapy with borderline patients. In N. Slavinska-Holy (Ed.), *Contemporary perspectives in group psychotherapy.* London: Routledge & Kegan Paul.

Stone, W., & Whiteman, R. (1980). Observation and empathy in group psychotherapy. In L. Wolberg & M. Aronson (Eds.), *Group and family therapy.* New York: Brunner/Mazel.

Stravynski, A., Grey, S., & Elie, R. (1987). Outline of the therapeutic process in social skills training with socially dysfunctional patients. *Journal of Consulting and Clinical Psychology,* 55, 224–228.

Stravynski, A., Marks, I., & Yule, W, (1982). Social skills problems in neurotic outpatients. *Archives of General Psychiatry,* 39, 1378–1383.

Stricker, G. (1983). Passive-aggressiveness: A condition especially suited to the psychodynamic approach. In R. Parsons & R. Wicks (Eds.), *Passive-aggressiveness: Theory and practice.* New York: Brunner/Mazel.

Strupp, H., & Binder, J. (1984). *Psychotherapy in a new key: A guide to time-limited dynamic psychotherapy.* New York: Basic Books.

Swiercinsky, D. (Ed.). (1985). *Testing adults.* Kansas City, MO: Test Corp. of America.

Symington, N. (1980). The response aroused by the psychopath. *International Review of Psychoanalysis,* 7, 291–298.

Tacbacnik, N. (1965). Isolation, transference, splitting and combined treatment. *Comprehensive Psychiatry,* 6, 336–346.

Thomas, A., & Chess, S. (1977). *Temperament and development.* New York: Brunner/Mazel.

Toman, W. (1961). *Family constellation: Theory and practice of a psychological game.* New York: Springer.

Torgerson, S. (1984). Genetic and nosological aspects of schizotypal and borderline personality disorders. *Archives of General Psychiatry,* 41, 546–554.

Turkat, I. (1985). Formulations of paranoid personality disorders. In I. Turkat (Ed.), *Behavioral case formulations.* New York: Plenum, pp. 161–198.

Turkat, I. (1986). The behavioral interview. In R. Ciminero, K. Calhoun, & H. Adams (Eds.), *Handbook of behavioral assessment* (2nd ed.). New York: Wiley-Interscience, pp. 109–149.

Turkat, I. (1990). *The personality disorders: A psychological approach to clinical management*. New York: Pergamon.

Turkat, I., & Banks, D. (1987). Paranoid personality and its disorder. *Journal of Psychopathology and Behavioral Assessment, 9*, 295–304.

Turkat, I., & Maisto, S. (1985). Application of the experimental method to the formulation and modification of personality disorders. In D. Barlow (Ed.), *Clinical handbook of psychological disorders*. New York: Guilford Press, pp. 503–570.

Turner, S., Beidel, D., & Burden, J. (1991). Social phobia: Axis I and II correlates. *Journal of Abnormal Psychology, 100*, 102–106.

Turner, S., Beidel, D., Dancu, C., et al. (1986). Psychopharmacology of social phobia and comparison to avoidant personality disorder. *Journal of Abnormal Psychology, 95*, 389–394.

Vaccani, J. (1989). Borderline personality and alcohol abuse. *Archives of Psychiatric Nursing, 3*, 113–119.

Vaillant, G., & Perry, J. (1985). Personality disorders. In H. Kaplan & B. Sadock (Eds.), *Comprehensive textbook of psychiatry* (4th ed.). Baltimore: Williams & Wilkins.

Veith, I. (1977). Four thousand years of hysteria. In M. Horowitz (Ed.), *Hysterical personality*. New York: Jason Aronson, pp. 7–23.

Vinogradov, S., & Yalom, I. (1989). *Concise guide to group psychotherapy*. Washington, DC: American Psychiatric Press.

Wagner, E., & Wagner, C. (1981). *The interpretation of psychological test data*. Springfield, IL: Charles C Thomas.

Waldinger, R. (1986). Intensive psychodynamic psychotherapy with borderline patients: An overview. *American Journal of Psychiatry, 144*, 267–274.

Waldo, M., & Harman, M. (1993). Relationship enhancement therapy with borderline personality. *Family Journal, 1*, 25–30.

Walker, R. (1992). Substance abuse and B-cluster disorders: Treatment recommendations. *Journal of Psychoactive Drugs, 24*, 233–241.

Wallerstein, R. (1986). *Forty-two lives in treatment. A study of psychoanalysis and psychotherapy*. New York: Guilford Press.

Weeks, G., & L'Abate, L. (1982). *Paradoxical psychotherapy: Theory and practice with individuals, couples, and families*. New York: Brunner/Mazel.

Wells, M., Glickhauf-Hughes, C., & Buzzel, V. (1990). Treating obsessive-compulsive personalities in psychoanalytic/interpersonal group therapy. *Psychotherapy, 27*, 366–379.

Wetzel, J. (1984). *Clinical handbook of depression*. New York: Gardner Press.

Wetzler, S. (1992). *Living with the passive-aggressive man*. New York: Simon & Schuster.

Widiger, T., & Corbitt, E. (1993). Antisocial personality disorder: Proposals for DSM-IV. *Journal of Personality Disorders, 7*, 63–77.

Williams, J. (1988). Cognitive intervention for a paranoid personality disorder. *Psychotherapy, 25*, 570–575.

Winer, J., & Pollock, G. (1989). Psychoanalytics and dynamic psychotherapy. In T. Karasu (Ed.), *Treatment of psychiatric disorders*. Washington, DC: American Psychiatric Press, pp. 2639–2648.

Winston, A., & Pollack, J. (1991). Brief adaptive psychotherapy. *Psychiatric Annals, 21*, 415–418.

Woody, G., McLellan, T., Luborsky, L., O'Brien, C. (1985). Sociopathy and psychotherapy outcome. *Archives of General Psychiatry, 42*, 1081–1086.

Wurmser, L. (1981). *The mask of shame*. Baltimore: Johns Hopkins University Press.

Yalom, I. (1985). *The theory and practice of group psychotherapy*. New York: Basic Books.

Young, P. (1990). *Cognitive therapy for personality disorders: A schema-focused approach*. Sarasota, FL: Professional Resource Exchange.

Yudofsky, S., William, D., & Gorman, J. (1981). Propranolol in treatment of rage and violent behavior in patients with chronic brain syndrome. *American Journal of Psychiatry, 38*, 218–220.

Zimbardo, P. (1977). *Shyness*. New York: Jove/Berkeley Publishing Group.

Zimmerman, M. (1994). Diagnosing personality disorders. *Archives of General Psychiatry, 51*, 225–245.

Zung, W. (1965). A self-rating depression scale. *Archives of General Psychiatry, 12*, 63–70.

Name Index

Abraham, 208
Abrams, G., 110
Abramson, R., 130
Adler, A., 13, 146, 179, 189
Adler, G., 56, 59, 66
Adler, L., 50–51
Akhtar, S., 155, 176
Akiskal, H., 205
Alden, L., 47–48, 50
Alexander, J., 31, 32, 89
Alonso, A., 128, 151
American Psychiatric Association, 19, 38, 58, 81, 100, 117, 139, 158, 195, 211
Andersen, J., 205
Anderson, C., 187
Antonuccio, D., 3
Appel, G., 185
Arieti, S., 2
Armstrong, H., 71, 72–73
Atterman, A., 27
Azima, F., 48, 185

Baer, L., 146
Baker, J., 82
Balint, E., 167
Balint, M., 167, 176
Banks, D., 160
Barlow, D., 93, 94
Barnes, R., 188
Beck, A., ix, 2, 3, 5, 13, 21, 28–29, 39, 45, 50, 51, 60, 69, 82, 89, 101, 118–119, 126, 127, 132, 141–142, 148, 159, 167, 178, 184, 185, 196, 202, 203, 213, 220

Beidel, D., 48, 145
Beitman, B., 3
Bellak, L., 2, 26, 65, 86, 105, 122, 145, 165, 182
Benjamin, L., ix, 5, 6, 13, 22, 29–30, 39–40, 46–47, 49, 61, 70, 83, 90–91, 101–102, 108–109, 119, 127, 142, 149–150, 160, 169–170, 172, 179, 185, 197, 203–204, 214, 221–222
Berger, P., 76
Berkowitz, D., 128, 129
Berman, E., 110
Bernstein, D., 154, 173, 191
Binder, J., 50, 87, 89, 125
Blackwell, B., 2, 12
Bleuler, 173, 208
Blum, N., 135
Bogdanoff, M., 186
Bohn, M., 25
Bomperad, J., 2
Bonime, W., 183
Boyd, J., 32
Buie, D., 66
Burden, J., 145
Burke, J., 32
Burke, W., 32
Burns, D., 209, 213, 223
Burry, A., 100, 102, 159, 177, 194
Buzzel, V., 150, 151, 153

Calabrese, J., 75, 205
Carlson, J., 179, 186, 189, 223
Carnegie, D., 202

239

Subject Index

245